Ultrasound technique videos – the perfect supplement!

Dynamic video sequences, in which doctors perform ultrasound scans of abdominal organs and vessels, on MediaCenter.thieme.com supplement the *Ultrasound Teaching Manual,* giving you the opportunity to view the examination techniques in detail. The sequences are short (each about 2–5 minutes) to maximize their impact and make it easier to retain the material. The videos are divided into the following sections:

I. **Introduction for beginners.**
A brief demonstration of the systematic approach and examination sequence on an anatomic poster, covering:
- Retroperitoneum
- Porta hepatis
- Liver
- Gallbladder
- Kidneys
- Spleen
- Bladder
- Orientation in the female pelvis
- FAST
- Thyroid gland

II. **Handling the transducer.**
Precise examination sequences and tips for transducer positioning, covering:
- General introduction to transducer positioning
- Retroperitoneum
- Porta hepatis
- Liver
- Gallbladder
- Right kidney
- Left kidney
- Spleen
- Bladder
- FAST
- Thyroid gland

III. **Transducer positioning and resulting ultrasound images.**
Synchronized detailed explanations of scanning procedures of:
- Retroperitoneum
- Porta hepatis
- Liver
- Gallbladder
- Right kidney
- Left kidney
- Spleen
- Bladder
- Orientation in the female pelvis
- FAST
- Thyroid gland

System requirements on next page.

D1344565

Simply visit MediaCenter.thieme.com, **and when prompted during the registration process, enter the scratch-off code below to get started.**

This book cannot be returned once this panel has been scratched off.

Find us on Facebook   *Connect with us on Facebook® for exclusive offers.*

	WINDOWS	MAC	TABLET
Recommended Browser(s) **	Microsoft Internet Explorer 8.0 or later, Firefox 3.x	Firefox 3.x, Safari 4.x	HTML5 mobile browser. iPad — Safari. Opera Mobile — Tablet PCs preferred.
	** *all browsers should have JavaScript enabled*		
Flash Player Plug-in	Flash Player 9 or Higher* * *Mac users: ATI Rage 128 GPU does not support full-screen mode with hardware scaling*		Tablet PCs with Android OS support Flash 10.1
Minimum Hardware Configurations	Intel® Pentium® II 450 MHz, AMD Athlon™ 600 MHz or faster processor (or equivalent) 512 MB of RAM	PowerPC® G3 500 MHz or faster processor Intel Core™ Duo 1.33 GHz or faster processor 512MB of RAM	Minimum CPU powered at 800MHz 256MB DDR2 of RAM
Recommended for optimal usage experience	Monitor resolutions: • Normal (4:3) 1024×768 or Higher • Widescreen (16:9) 1280×720 or Higher • Widescreen (16:10) 1440×900 or Higher DSL/Cable internet connection at a minimum speed of 384.0 Kbps or faster WiFi 802.11 b/g preferred.		7-inch and 10-inch tablets on maximum resolution. WiFi connection is required.

BMA

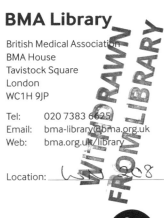

Ultrasound Teaching Manual

An Introductory Workbook

Third expanded and revised English edition

Matthias Hofer

782 figures and 43 tables

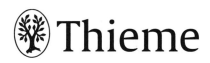 Thieme

Matthias Hofer, MD, MPH, MME (University of Bern)
Diagnostic Radiologist
Head, Medical Education Pilot Project
Heinrich Heine University
P.O. Box 10 10 07
40001 Düsseldorf, Germany

With gynecologic images contributed by:
Tatjana Reihs, MD
Dept. of Obstetrics and Gynecology
Heinrich Heine University
P.O. Box 10 10 07
40001 Düsseldorf, Germany

1st German edition 1995
1st Japanese edition 1995
1st Dutch edition 1996
2nd German edition 1997
1st Greek edition 1997
1st English edition 1999
3rd German edition 1999
2nd Japanese edition 2000
1st French edition 2001
1st Italian edition 2001
4th German edition 2002
1st Portuguese edition 2003
1st Russian edition 2003
1st Spanish edition 2004
1st Czech edition 2005
2nd English edition 2005
5th German edition 2005
2nd Italian edition 2006
2nd Spanish edition 2007
2nd Greek edition 2008
1st Polish edition 2008
6th German edition 2009
7th German edition 2012
3rd Italian edition 2012

© 2013 Thieme Publishers, Stuttgart, New York
Home page: http://www.thieme.de
Printed in Germany

Design: Susanne Kniest, Kaarst
3rd English edition:
Inger Wollziefer, Berlin, www.designinger.de
Front-/ Backcover: Thieme Publishers
Printing: Druckerei Steinmeier, Deiningen

ISBN   9783131110435
eISBN 9783131734433

Bibliographic information of the German National Library

The German National Library lists this publication in the German National Bibliography; detailed bibliographical data are available on the Internet at http://dnb.ddb.de.

Important note:

Like every science, medicine is undergoing continuous development. Research and clinical experience are continuously expanding our knowledge, in particular our knowledge of proper treatment and drug therapy. Insofar as this book mentions any dosage or application, readers may rest assured that the author and publisher have made every effort to ensure that such references are in accordance with **the state of knowledge at the time of production of the book.**

Nevertheless, this does not involve, imply, or express any guarantee on the part of the publisher with respect to any dosage instructions and forms of application stated in the book. **Every user is requested to examine carefully** the manufacturer's package inserts accompanying each drug and to check, if necessary in consultation with a specialist, whether the dosage schedules mentioned therein or the contraindications stated by the manufacturers differ from the statements made in the present book. Such examination is particularly important with drugs that are either rarely used or have been newly released on the market. **Every dosage schedule or every form of application used is entirely at the user's own risk. The user assumes sole responsibility for every diagnostic and therapeutic application, medication, and dosage.** Consequently, the author and publisher assume no responsibility and no liability whatsoever for any damages of any sort that may occur as a result of use of information, in whole or in part, contained in the present book. We request every user to report to the publisher any discrepancies or inaccuracies noticed.

How can you use this workbook optimally?

As you work through the individual chapters, you can benefit from several methodical and didactic features:

Find it quickly ...

- Find a chapter: you will find the respective tab for each chapter on page 5.
- Find tough quiz questions for in-depth study, also explained on page 5.
- Find cross-referenced figures: the figures are numbered according to the page on which they appear. For example, **Fig. 36.2** is on page 36.
- Find an explanatory figure or diagram supplementing the text. They are highlighted in light blue in the accompanying text and are almost always on the same page, eliminating the need to page through the book looking for them.
- Find numbered structures. Their reference numbers appear in bold in the accompanying text or on the back cover flap (the same number is used throughout the entire book).
- Find keywords on page 121 (or on pages 4 and 5).

- Find normal values and checklists. These are also provided on laminated, water-resistant, pocket-sized cards.

Why is this book called a "workbook"?

A unique feature of this book is that you can use every page as a quiz to test your knowledge. The diagrams contain reference numbers instead of labels. This means you can go through the material a second time and use any figure to test which structures you know and which still have to learn. The quiz questions and drawing exercises have a similar purpose.

In this way, you can become familiar with several efficient study methods that allow you to integrate new material into your long-term memory faster – even though this requires you to take a more active approach to learning. Not only do I wish you good luck with this course, I also hope you have fun doing it!

Matthias Hofer, MD, MME, October 2012

List of Abbreviations

A.	Artery	ESWL	Extracorporeal shock wave lithotripsy	MRI	Magnetic resonance imaging
Aa.	Arteries			mW	Milliwatt
AC	Abdominal circumference (fetus)	FL	Femur length (fetus)	NHL	Non-Hodgkin lymphoma
AG	Adrenal gland	FNH	Focal nodular hyperplasia	NT	Nuchal translucency (fetus)
AIUM	American Institute of Ultrasound in Medicine	FOD	Fronto-occipital diameter (fetus)	PP	Parenchyma-pelvis (index)
		GI	Gastrointestinal	PT	Preterm newborn
AO	Aorta	HC	Head circumference	PW	Pulsed wave (Doppler)
ASD	Atrial septal defect	HCG	Human chorionic gonadotropin	RI	Resistive index
BPD	Biparietal diameter (fetus)	IHW	Width of the SAS in the interhemispheric fissure	RT	Renal transplant
b/w	Black-white (B-mode) ultrasound			SAS	Subarachnoid space
CCD	Chorionic cavity diameter	IUD	Intrauterine device	SCW	Sinocortical width of the SAS
CCE	Cholecystectomy	IVC	Inferior vena cava	SD	Standard deviation
CCW	Craniocerebral width of the external subarachnoid space	IVF	In vitro fertilization	SLE	Systemic lupus erythematosus
		IVP	Intravenous pyelogram	SMA	Superior mesenteric artery
CHI	Contrast harmonic imaging	LA	Lower abdomen	TGA	Transposition of the great arteries
CRL	Crown–rump length (fetus)	Lig.	Ligament	THI	Tissue harmonic imaging
CSF	Cerebrospinal fluid	LN	Lymph node	UA	Upper abdomen
CT	Computed tomography	M.	Muscle	V.	Vein
CW	Continuous wave (Doppler)	MA	Mid-abdomen	Vv.	Veins
d_{Ao}	Diameter of the aorta	MCL	Midclavicular line	VSD	Ventricular septal defect
DGC	Depth gain compensation	MCU	Micturating cystourethrogram = voiding cystourethrogram	YS	Yolk sac
d_{VC}	Diameter of the vena cava				
ERCP	Endoscopic retrograde cholangiopancreatography	MHz	Megahertz (unit of frequency)		
		Mm.	Muscles		

Contents

Standard Planes   (front cover flap)

Physical Principles and Technique
Image Formation: Sound Transmission, Reflection	6
Echogenicity, Frequency Ranges	7
Operation and Specification of an Ultrasound Unit	8
Selection of Ultrasound Units, Types of Transducers	9

New Techniques
Panoramic Imaging, 3D, Clarify Vascular Enhancement	10
Harmonic Imaging	11
Phase Inversion, Contrast Enhancement	12
SonoCT	13
Pulse Compression, Precision Up-Sampling	14
Diagnostic Ultrasound Catheter	15

Artifacts
Reverberation, Section Thickness, Distal Acoustic Enhancement	16
Acoustic Shadowing, Mirror Image	17
Side Lobe Artifact, Quiz for Self Evaluation	18

Practical Tips and Tricks for the Beginner   19

Lesson 1   Abdomen

Retroperitoneum, Sagittal Plane
Upper Retroperitoneum, Normal Findings	21
Lower Retroperitoneum, Normal Findings	22
Aortic Ectasia and Aneurysms	23
Retroperitoneal Lymph Nodes	24
Other Clinical Cases, Right Heart Failure	25
Quiz for Self Evaluation	26

Lesson 2   Abdomen

Transverse Planes of the Upper Abdomen, Pancreas
Basic Anatomy	27
Normal Findings	28
Acute and Chronic Pancreatitis, Age-related Echogenicity	29
Pancreas: Other Cases	30
Lymph Nodes	31
Porta Hepatis: Normal Findings	32
Porta Hepatis: Portal Hypertension, Lymph Nodes	33
Quiz for Self Evaluation	34

Lesson 3   Abdomen

Liver
Organ Size, Lateral Angle, Gallbladder	35
Hepatic Venous Star, Right Heart Failure	36
Normal Variants, Fatty Liver	37
Focal Fatty Infiltration	38
Cysts, Parasites, and Hemangiomas	39
Other Focal Hepatic Lesions, Air in the Bile Ducts	40
Cirrhosis and Hepatocellular Carcinoma	41
Liver Metastases, Quiz Question	42

Gallbladder and Bile Ducts
Bile Ducts: Cholestasis	43
Gallstones and Polyps	44
Gallbladder: Cholecystitis	45
Liver and Gallbladder: Quiz for Self Evaluation	46

Lesson 4   Abdomen

Kidney
Normal Findings	47
Normal Variants and Cysts	48
Kidneys and Urinary System in Pediatrics:	
Normal Findings	49
Changes in the Renal Parenchyma	50
Degeneration and Inflammation	51
Urinary Obstruction	52
Differential Diagnosis of Urinary Obstruction	53
Urinary Obstruction and Reflux in Pediatrics	54
Voiding Cystourethrogram	55
Kidney Stones and Infarcts	56
Renal and Adrenal Tumors	57
Renal and Adrenal Tumors in Pediatrics	58

Bladder
Normal Findings	59
Indwelling Catheter and Cystitis	60
Bladder in Pediatrics	61

Renal Transplants (RT)
Normal Findings	62
Complications	63
Quiz for Self Evaluation	64

Lesson 5   Abdomen

Gastrointestinal Tract
Stomach	65
Small Bowel: Crohn Disease, Ascites, Hernias	67
Gastrointestinal Tract in Children: Intussusception, Contrast Enema	68
Appendicitis, Diarrhea, Hirschsprung Disease	69
Colon: Fecal Impaction, Colitis, Diverticulitis	70

Spleen
Normal Findings, Curtain Trick	71
Diffuse Splenomegaly, Systemic Hematologic Disorders	72
Focal Lesions: Infarcts, Lymphomatous Infiltration, Other Lesions	73
Size Measurements, Quiz for Self Evaluation	74

Lesson 6   Reproductive Organs

Male Reproductive Organs
Prostate Gland, Prostatic Hypertrophy, Testes and Scrotum	75
Undescended Testis, Orchitis, Epididymitis, Hydrocele, Inguinal Hernia	76

Female Reproductive Organs
Endovaginal Ultrasound, Image Orientation	77
Uterus: Normal Findings, Intrauterine Device	78
Uterine Tumors, Myoma, Adenocarcinoma	79
Ovaries: Normal Findings, Volume Measurement, Cycle Phases	80
Ovaries: Cysts, Tumors, Infertility Therapy	81
Pregnancy Testing, Ectopic Pregnancy	82
Placenta Position and Gender Determination	83
Biometry in the First Trimester: CCD, YSD, CRL	84
Biometry in the 2nd and 3rd Trimesters: BPD, FL, AC	85

Contents

Diagnosis of Malformations
Cerebellum and CSF Spaces — 86
Spine: Spinal Anatomy, Spina Bifida — 87
Facial Bones, Nuchal Translucency, Hydrops Fetalis — 88
Heart and Blood Vessels: Congenital Cardiac Shunts — 89
Gastrointestinal Tract, Omphalocele, Kidneys — 90
Bones of the Extremities: Clubfoot — 91
Reproductive Organs: Quiz for Self Evaluation — 92

Lesson 7   Head and Neck

Neonatal Skull
Normal Findings in the Coronal Plane — 93
CSF Spaces, Normal Findings in the Sagittal Plane — 95
Normal Variants: Cavum of the Septum Pellucidum, — 97
Agenesis of the Corpus Callosum
Hemorrhages: Pathophysiology, Ultrasound — 98
Morphology
Hydrocephalus, Cerebral Atrophy — 99
Monitoring the Shunt in Hydrocephalus, Spinal Canal — 100

Thyroid Gland
Normal Findings: Anatomy, Volumetric — 101
Measurements
Pathologic Cases: Goiter — 102
Focal Solid Nodules, Thyroiditis, Volumetric — 103
Measurements

Neck
Lymph Nodes, Differential Diagnostic Criteria — 104

Pediatrics: Hip
Preparation, Positioning the Newborn — 107
Ultrasound Documentation
Setup and Measurement Errors — 109
Classification of Infant Hips According to Graf — 110

Head and Neck: Quiz for Self Evaluation — 111

Emergency Diagnostics — 112
FAST: Focused Assessment with Sonography for
Trauma

Appendix
Diagram Templates for Standard Planes — 114
Primer of Ultrasound Findings — 116
Index — 120
Template for Report of Normal Ultrasound Findings — 121
Answers to the Questions — 122
Acknowledgments — 126
Information About Practical Ultrasound Courses — 126

Table of Normal Values for Adults   (back cover flap)
Table of Normal Values for Prenatal Care

Legend of numbered structures   (inner back cover flap)

Where Do I Find Which Chapter?

Physical Principles and Technique — 6

Lesson 1
Retroperitoneum — 21

Lesson 2
Transverse Planes of the UA, Pancreas — 27

Lesson 3
Liver, Gallbladder, Bile Ducts — 35

Lesson 4
Kidneys, Adrenal Glands, Bladder, RT — 47

Lesson 5
Gastrointestinal Tract, Spleen — 65

Lesson 6
Reproductive Organs, Malformations — 75

Images courtesy of Dr. Tatjana Reihs

Lesson 7
Head, Neck, Hip, and FAST — 93

Answers to Quiz Questions, — 116
Ultrasound Primer

Do you want to do more than "just read"?
Experience has shown that readers and course participants benefit most from this book by applying a little determination and learning to draw the standard planes from memory and solving the quiz questions by themselves. You will be surprised how much quicker you will integrate this new material into your long-term memory. To find the relevant pages more easily, the quiz headings are marked in blue in the table of contents and the pages are marked with a blue tab in the margin:

Q

Are you interested in pediatrics?
We have also introduced margin tabs to highlight pages with pediatric content. The tabs appear just above the lower corner of the outer edge of each page. The tabs look like this:
Pediatric material is found on pages 49, 50, 53–55, 58, 61, 65, 68, 69, 74, 93–100, 107–110.

P

Image Formation

Ultrasound images are generated not by X-rays but by sound waves that are sent by a transducer into the human body and reflected there. In abdominal ultrasound, the frequencies used generally are between 2.5 and 5.0 megahertz (MHz; see p. 9).

The primary condition required for sound wave reflections is the presence of so-called "impedance mismatches." These occur at the interface between two tissue layers with different sound transmission properties (interfaces in **Fig. 6.2**). It is interesting to note that different soft tissues show only minor differences in the transmission of sound (**Table 6.1**). Only air and bone are marked by massively different sound transmission in comparison with other human tissue.

For this reason ultrasound units can be operated at a preselected medium frequency of approximately 1540 m/s without producing any major inaccuracies in the calculated origin ("depth") of the echo. The processor computes the depth of origin of the echo from the time difference detected between emission of the sound impulse and return of the echo. Echoes from tissue close to the transducer (**A**) arrive earlier (t_A) than echoes from deeper tissues (t_B, t_C in **Fig. 6.2a**). The mean frequency is strictly theoretical since the processor cannot know which type of tissue was traversed.

Sound Transmission in Human Tissue		
Air	331 m/s	
Liver	1549 m/s	
Spleen	1566 m/s	mean = 1540 m/s
Muscle	1568 m/s	
Bone	3360 m/s	

Table 6.1

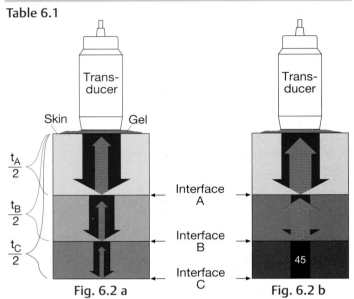

Fig. 6.2 a   Fig. 6.2 b

Which Component of the Sound Wave is Reflected?

Fig. 6.2a shows three tissue blocks traversed by sound waves that differ only minimally in their transmission velocity (indicated by similar gray values). Each interface only reflects a small portion of the original sound waves (↓) as echo (↑). The right–hand diagram shows a larger impedance mismatch at the interface A between the different tissues (**Fig. 6.2b**). This increases the proportion of reflected sound waves (↑) in comparison to the tissues shown on the left. However, what happens if the sound waves hit air in the stomach or a rib? This causes a so-called "total reflection," as illustrated at interface B (**Fig. 6.2b**). The transducer does not detect any residual sound waves deep to this structure from which it can generate an image. Instead, the total reflection creates an acoustic shadow (**45**).

Conclusion: Intestinal or pulmonary air and bone are impenetrable by sound waves, precluding any imaging deep to these structures. The goal will later be to work around intestinal air or ribs by maneuvering the transducer. The pressure applied to the transducer against the abdominal wall (see p. 19) and the acoustic gel that displaces air between the surface of the transducer and the patient's skin (see p. 20) play a significant role.

From a "Snowstorm" to an Image ...

Do not get discouraged if at first you can only make a blinding "snowstorm" on ultrasound images. You will be surprised how soon you will recognize the ultrasound morphology of individual organs and vessels. **Fig. 6.3** shows two round polyps (**65**) in the gallbladder (**14**), visualized as a black structure. The surrounding gray "snowstorm" corresponds to the hepatic parenchyma (**9**), which is traversed by hepatic vessels (**10, 11**). How can you quickly work out which structures in the image appear bright and which are dark? The key lies in the concept of echogenicity (see p. 7).

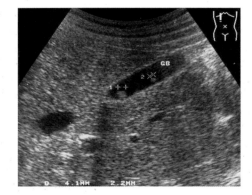

Fig. 6.3 a

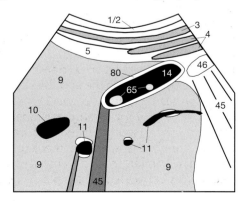

Fig. 6.3 b

What Does the Term "Echogenicity" Mean?

Tissues or organs with many intrinsic impedance mismatches produce many echoes and appear **"hyperechoic"** = bright. In contrast, tissue and organs with few impedance mismatches appear **"hypoechoic"** = dark. Consequently, homogeneous fluids without impedance mismatches (blood, urine, bile, cerebrospinal fluid, pericardial or pleural effusion, ascites, cyst secretion) appear **"anechoic"** = black.

The number of impedance mismatches does not depend on the physical density (= mass per unit of volume). This is best illustrated with a fatty liver.

Please use the following terms:	These appear an-echoic (= black):
Hyperechoic (= bright) **Hypoechoic (= dark)** **Anechoic (= black)**	Blood, urine, bile, cerebrospinal fluid, pericardial or pleural effusion, ascites, cysts

On this noncontrasted CT scan **(Fig. 7.1a)**, the parenchyma of a fatty liver **(9)** appears darker (i.e., less dense) than hepatic vessels or normal liver **(Fig. 7.1b)**. This is due to the lesser density of fat in comparison with normal liver tissue.

On ultrasound the fatty deposits produce more impedance mismatches **(Fig. 7.1c)** than in normal liver tissue **(Fig. 7.1d)**. Consequently, a fatty liver appears more echogenic (brighter) on ultrasound despite its significantly lower physical density.

A common misunderstanding:

What do ultrasound examiners mean when they refer to a "dense liver"? Either they are not expressing themselves clearly or they have failed to grasp the fundamental principle of ultrasound imaging and how it differs from radiography. Ultrasound does not visualize physical tissue densities but differences in sound transmission (impedance mismatches) which are unrelated to density.

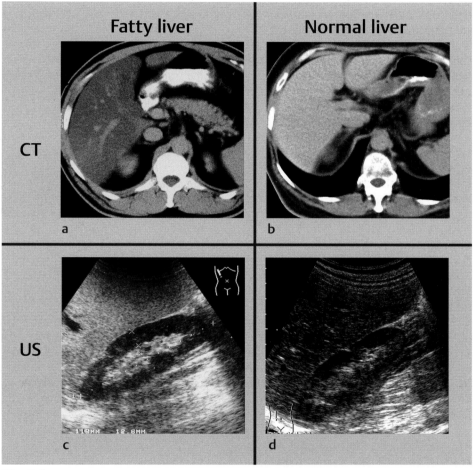

Fig. 7.1

Generation and Frequency Ranges of Sound Waves

Sound waves are generated by what is known as the "piezo-electric effect." The pressure waves of an echo distort crystals, causing them to emit an electrical impulse. The reverse takes place during transmission. A transducer includes many such crystals. Depending on the impulse applied, they can produce sound waves of various frequencies specified in megahertz (MHz). A "3.75–MHz" transducer does not exclusively emit pressure waves (sound waves) at a frequency of 3.75 MHz; that is merely the specified median frequency (= **"center frequency"**). In fact, such a transducer may emit sound wave frequencies between, for example, 2 and 6 MHz.

So-called **"multi-frequency transducers"** have the additional capability to increase or decrease this center frequency and the surrounding bandwidth of transmitted sound frequencies. In thin patients or children, for instance, the bandwidth can be shifted (say 4–8 MHz with a center frequency of 6 MHz) to achieve better spatial resolution. However, this decreases the depth penetration of the sound waves.

In very obese patients, the use of lower frequencies (1–5 MHz with a center frequency of 2.5 MHz) can be appropriate to achieve the necessary penetration, but at the cost lower resolution (see p. 9). Newer methods base their image generation on frequency shifts or harmonic frequencies of the echo in relation to the original ultrasound impulse (see p. 11).

Operating an Ultrasound Unit

Many controls on different ultrasound units are quite similar in function and arrangement regardless of the manufacturer. Therefore this section will look at the console of one unit, which will then be used to introduce common technical terms.

One common feature on almost all units is the freeze button (E) in the lower right corner of the console (Fig. 8.1). This freezes the moving image. It is recommended to rest one finger of your left hand lightly on the trackball or over this button during the examination to minimize delay in capturing a desired image.

Before you begin, do not forget to enter the patient's name (A, B) to eliminate any possible confusion in your imaging documentation later. The buttons for selecting a new menu (C) or transducer (D) are usually found at the top of the console. The menu function allows you to store predefined programs for specific examinations with optimized settings for frequency range, transducer type, penetration depth, etc. These programs make it easy to switch quickly between studies of different regions such as from an abdominal to a thyroid scan.

Fig. 8.1 Console and keyboard

A	Begin a new patient
B	Enter name (ID)
C	Change menu
D	Change transducer
E	Freeze
F	Gain
G	Depth gain compensation
H	Depth / range
I	Trackball for positioning markers or measuring points
J	Measurements
K	Comment
L	Body marker ("Where was the transducer placed?")
M	Image recording / printer

The overall amplification (gain) of the received echoes is usually controlled by a gain knob (F) that is normally a little larger than the other controls. The amplification of echoes can also be selectively adjusted with a series of sliding controls (G), each for a specific depth range. The better units allow fine incremental adjustment of the magnification or visualized depth (depth/range) as required (H).

It requires some practice to operate the trackball (I) with the left hand to take measurements or set markers. In general, this must be preceded by activating one of the measurement programs (J) or the comment mode (K). To make review of the images easier for others, the appropriate body marker (L) can be selected to mark the position of the transducer on the image before printing (M). The remaining functions vary among the different manufacturers and are best learned in clinical practice.

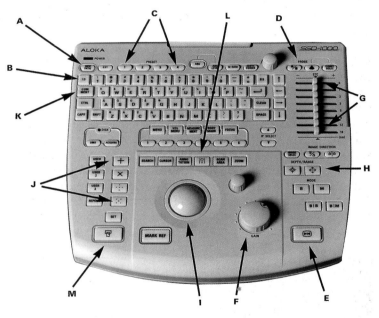

Specification of an Ultrasound Unit

Aside from price and image quality, you should carefully evaluate the user friendliness. For example, small units may have only one transducer plug. This can later become rather annoying when different types of transducers are often required (see p. 9).

In view of the increasing digitalization in hospitals and physician's offices, it is advisable to test the new unit for several days for compatibility with the existing data storage system. Unexpected problems invariably arise or are revealed within the scope of the supplier's customer service. Resolving them up front avoids subsequent disappointments or time-consuming or costly upgrades. To create a patient-friendly environment it is advisable to install a second monitor in the field of view of the supine patient, for instance beneath the ceiling. This will allow you to explain findings during the study. This additional investment can improve the doctor–patient relationship and enhance the reputation of your practice or hospital.

Although they probably stand to gain the most, pediatricians are not the only ones to benefit from a unit with digital storage (cine loop) of sufficient capacity to allow flashbacks for two or more seconds after freezing. This option allows one to record optimal images and use them for measurements even in restless patients (or where the image was frozen too late) without having to repeat the examination. This option is now also available even in smaller B-mode units.

Selection of Ultrasound Units

In addition to large color Doppler units, ultrasound units with connections for several multi-frequency transducers have proven especially useful in a hospital setting. Such mobile units are easily moved from the ultrasound suite to the ward or intensive care unit (**Fig. 9.1**).

The most important precaution when transporting the unit is to make sure that transducers are safely stowed so that dangling cables cannot become caught on doorknobs, gurneys, etc. A transducer that falls on the floor can easily represent a loss of €5000–10,000 ($6400–12,800) depending on the model. For the same reason, the transducer should never be left unattended on the patient's abdomen when the examination is interrupted, for instance by a telephone call. Stowing the transducer in the frame with the cable hanging avoids unnecessary kinking that can lead to broken conductors in the cable.

Types of Transducers

Of the many types of transducers, only the three most important ones will be discussed here (endovaginal transducers, see p. 77).

A **linear array transducer** emits parallel sound waves into the tissue and produces a rectangular image (**Fig. 9.2a**). The width of the image and the number of scan lines remain constant at all tissue levels. Linear array transducers have the advantage of good near-field resolution and are primarily used with high frequencies (5.0–10.0 MHz or higher) for evaluating soft tissue and the thyroid gland. Their disadvantage is the large contact surface. This can lead to air gaps between skin and transducer when it is applied to a curved body contour. Furthermore, acoustic shadowing (45) caused by ribs, lungs, or intestinal air can greatly degrade image quality. Conse-

quently, linear array transducers are rarely used for visualizing thoracic or abdominal organs.

A **sector transducer** produces a fanlike image that is narrow near the transducer and increases in width with deeper penetration (**Fig. 9.2b**). This type of transducer has become established primarily in cardiology with lower frequencies (2.0–3.0 MHz) allowing deeper penetration. Due to the fanlike propagation of the sound waves, the heart can be well visualized through a small intercostal window without acoustic shadows from the ribs. The disadvantages of this type of transducer are their poor near-field resolution and decreasing line density in the far field with correspondingly decreasing resolution. Moreover, finding the desired imaging plane is difficult and takes some practice.

The **curved or convex array transducer** is a combination of the two types described above (**Fig. 9.2c**). The shape of the monitor image resembles a coffee filter and combines good near-field resolution with relatively good far-field resolution. The major advantage of the slightly curved contact surface is its ability to displace interfering intestinal air outside the imaging plane (see p. 19). With this type of transducer, however, one has to accept decreasing resolution with increasing depth and, in certain locations, acoustic shadowing behind the ribs. This type is usually used in abdominal ultrasound with frequencies from 2.5 MHz (in very obese patients) to 5.0 MHz (in slender patients). The average frequency (center frequency) is usually 3.5–3.75 MHz. **Memory aid:** The higher the frequency, the better the resolution and the worse the penetration. The best way to remember this is to compare it to that annoying loud music from your neighbor's apartment. Which tones best penetrate even thick walls? The basses. These lower frequencies travel farther (i.e., penetrate deeper), see page 7.

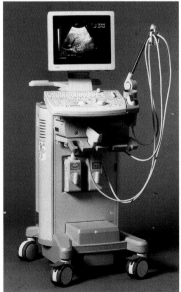

Fig. 9.1

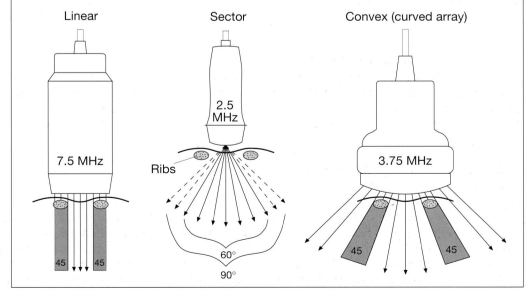

Fig. 9.2 a   Fig. 9.2 b   Fig. 9.2 c

Panoramic Imaging (SieScape®)

High-performance image processors generate extensive ultrasound images from data acquired as the examiner moves the transducer slowly and continuously over the region of interest. With some practice, the examiner can produce impressive and undistorted images that allow distance measurements accurate to within 1–3% even on a curved body surface. **Fig. 10.1** shows a sagittal scan with massive pleural effusion (69),

compressive atelectasis of the lung (47), and anechoic ascites (68) inferior to the liver (9) and inundating the small bowel (46).

Fig. 10.2 impressively illustrates the position of the placenta (94) relative to the fetus. The high contrast resolution even allows evaluation of the interface between the fetal liver (9) and lung (47).

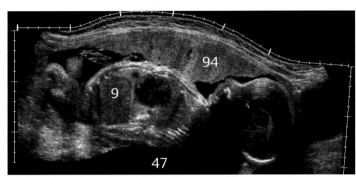

Fig. 10.1   **Fig. 10.2**

(With kind permission of Drs. C.F. Dietrich and D. Becker, from *Farbduplexsonographie des Abdomens*, Schnetzler-Verlag, Konstanz, Germany.)

3-D Visualization

Especially in obstetrics, the three-dimensional visualization of fetal facial features improves the diagnosis of malformations such as cleft lip and palate. This technique can now visualize the fetal physiognomy with amazing accuracy (**Fig. 10.3**).

Of course, conventional cross-sectional imaging techniques can also detect skeletal and other malformations (see p. 91), albeit less impressively and clearly than three-dimensional visualization.

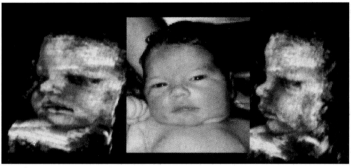

Fig. 10.3 (Wolfgang Krzos, Siemens)

Clarify Vascular Enhancement Technology

This technique is based on an algorithm that is able to significantly reduce the blurring on B-mode scans resulting from partial volume or section thickness artifacts. Flow information from the power Doppler mode is used, which helps to improve the spatial resolution of vascular contours on the B-mode image.

The result is significantly improved visualization of findings such as the contours of hard and soft plaque in the carotid arteries (**Fig. 10.4b**) compared with the visualization achieved by the conventional technique shown in **Fig. 10.4a**. It also facilitates evaluation of peripheral vascular rarefaction in the liver as the lumens of the hepatic veins and portal venous branches are more clearly visualized in the hepatic parenchyma (**Fig. 10.5**).

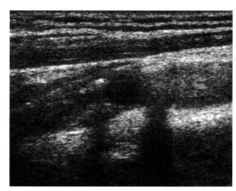
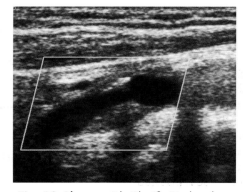
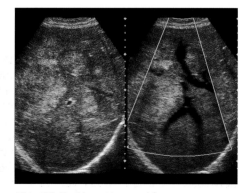

Fig. 10.4a "Normal" image of the carotid artery

Fig. 10.4b ... with Clarify Technology

Fig. 10.5 Hepatic vessels

The material on the following six pages is not an absolute prerequisite for the first practice sessions and can be skipped. Beginners may prefer to move from here directly to Lesson 1 (see p. 19). After some initial practice they should return to these pages to reinforce their fundamental understanding of ultrasound imaging.

Tissue Harmonic Imaging

This technique does not use the fundamental frequency of the original ultrasound impulse but their harmonics (integer multiples of the fundamental frequency), for example 7.0 MHz for a fundamental frequency of 3.5 MHz. These harmonics increase with increasing penetration, but their amplitude (intensity) remains far less than that of the base signal. The advantage of these harmonics is that they hardly arise at all near the transducer, but develop with increasing penetra-

tion depth (**Fig. 11.1**). Consequently, they are less affected by the major sources of scattered image noise. Why do harmonics develop only with increasing penetration depth?

Ultrasound waves are distorted as they traverse tissues with varying acoustic properties. Their pressure waves compress and relax the tissue as they penetrate it. Compressed tissue increases the speed of sound, whereas relaxed tissue decreases the speed and causes the trough of the pressure wave to propagate more slowly. The resulting distortion of the wave form (**Fig. 11.2**) induces harmonics. This is a cumulative effect that increases with the depth of penetration. Consequently, the amplitudes of the harmonic frequencies initially increase with penetration depth until this increase is offset by general absorption (**Fig. 11.1**).

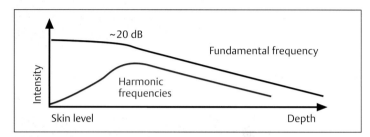

Fig. 11.1

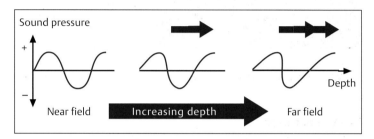

Fig. 11.2

Second Harmonic Imaging

This technique uses only the doubled frequency of the base signal for imaging. To avoid any overlapping of the range of the fundamental frequency (**Fig. 11.3a**) a narrow-band signal must be used to distinguish the stronger components of the fundamental frequency from the weaker components of the harmonic. However, the narrower bandwidth of the signal

leads to a slight reduction in contrast and spatial resolution. In spite of these shortcomings, this technique has markedly improved the detection of details (**Fig. 11.4b**) compared with conventional ultrasound imaging (**Fig. 11.4a**), especially in obese patients (whose abdominal wall produces excessive scattering).

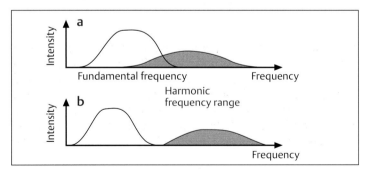

Fig. 11.3

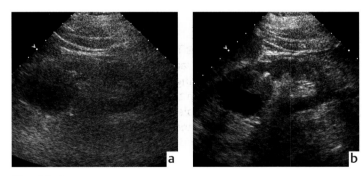

Fig. 11.4

Phase Inversion Technique

A broadband technique has since become established that allows the use of dynamically optimized harmonic multiples of the transmitted frequency with a broader bandwidth (Ensemble® THI, **Fig. 12.1c**). With this technique, image optimization no longer depends on the narrow bandwidth of the fundamental frequency (**Fig. 12.1a**) to cleanly separate it from its harmonics (**Fig. 12.1b**). Two successive pulses are transmitted in such a way that the phase (upward excursion of the pressure = positive, downward excursion = negative) of the second pulse is inverted to the phase of the first pulse (**Fig. 11.5**).

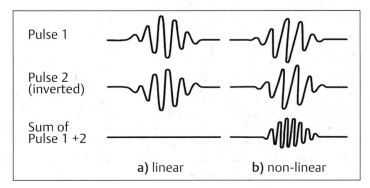

Fig. 11.5

If the echoes of both signals are added, the sum equals zero as long as the signal has **not** undergone any changes in the body. As a result, both fundamental frequency echoes are suppressed (**Fig. 11.5a**) whereas the second harmonic signal components are enhanced (**Fig. 11.5b**). **Fig. 12.2** depicts a case showing acoustic shadowing (↑ ↑ ↑) deep to intra-renal calcifications (**b**) that are undetectable by conventional imaging (**a**). In addition, the renal cyst (↘) appears better demarcated and can be classified as benign with greater confidence.

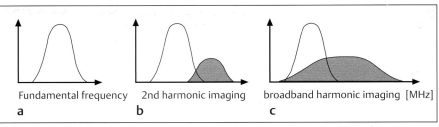

Fig. 12.1

Contrast Enhancement

The echogenicity of blood and tissue can be enhanced with microbubbles with a diameter of 3–5 µm that pass through the capillaries and change the impedance within the blood stream (**Fig. 12.3**). So far, several contrast enhancement agents have been introduced and about 50 additional agents are under development.

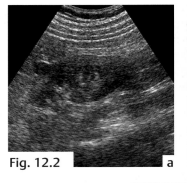

Fig. 12.2   **a**   **b**

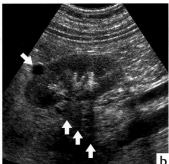

The contrast agent **Leovist**® consists of tiny air bubbles (∗) about 3 µm in diameter (95% < 10 µm), which are stabilized with a thin envelope of palmitic acid (**Fig. 12.4**). They are initially bound to galactose microparticles that dissolve in the blood and release the microbubbles. The dry powder can be mixed by the examiner in different concentrations. The suspension passes through the pulmonary circulation, but is only injectable for about 8 minutes after preparation. Hypergalactosemia is a contraindication.

The contrast agent **Optison**® consists of octafluoropropane microbubbles with human serum albumin as an adjuvant. Until now it has primarily been used in cardiology. The mean size of the microbubbles is about 3.7 µm (shown in **Fig. 12.5** in comparison with erythrocytes). The octafluoropropane is almost completely eliminated by the lungs within about 10 minutes of administration. Any possible virus contamination of the serum albumin is inactivated by plasma fractionation with 40% alcohol and by pasteurization at 60°C for 10 hours.

The contrast agent **Sonovue**® consists of an aqueous solution of sulfur hexafluoride (SF6) stabilized by a phospholipid layer (**Fig. 12.6**). The median size of the bubbles is about 2.5 µm (90% < 8 µm) with an osmolality of 290 mOsmol/kg. One possible advantage of this contrast agent is that the suspension remains stable for over 6 hours, allowing it to be used for several successive applications.

The best results are achieved in conjunction with the tissue harmonic imaging (THI) technique, referred to as **"contrast harmonic imaging (CHI)."** A specific sound pressure causes the bubbles to vibrate and emit harmonic echoes. As a result, contrast harmonic imaging can significantly better detect multiple liver metastases (**Fig. 12.7b**) than noncontrasted imaging (**Fig. 12.7a**).

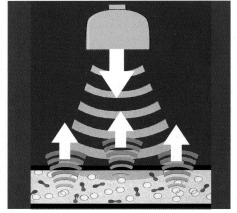

Fig. 12.3

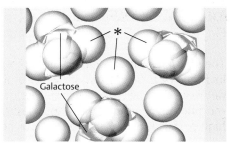

Fig. 12.4

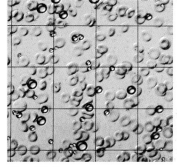

Fig. 12.5

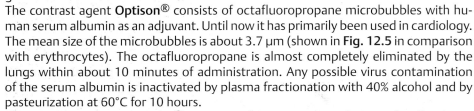

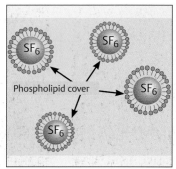

Fig. 12.6

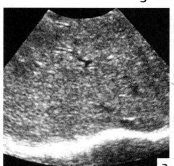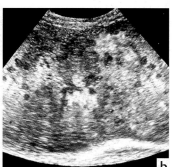

Fig. 12.7   **a**   **b**

Spatial Compounding (SonoCT®)

There is another technique for suppressing artifacts. "Real-time compound imaging" does not scan an image line by line (Fig. 13.1a), instead it scans from different angles and merges this data into an image in real time (Fig. 13.1b). Up to nine slices can be scanned, allowing more precise visualization of tissue information. This is illustrated here by the morphology of arteriosclerotic plaque in the carotid artery (Fig. 13.2a) compared with conventional imaging (Fig. 13.2b).

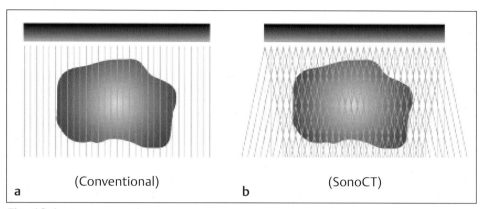

(Conventional)   (SonoCT)

a   b

Fig. 13.1

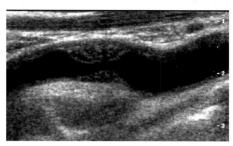

Fig. 13.2 a

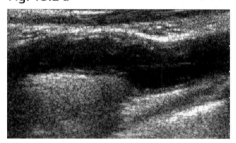

Fig. 13.2 b

This technique has exhibited obvious advantages in ultrasound imaging of the breast and musculoskeletal system. **Fig. 13.3b** shows improved visualization of an entire biopsy needle (➘) in the breast parenchyma in comparison with conventional imaging (**Fig. 13.3a**), allowing more precise localization of the suspicious lesion.

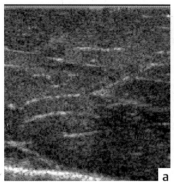 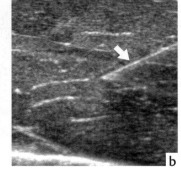

a   b

Fig. 13.3

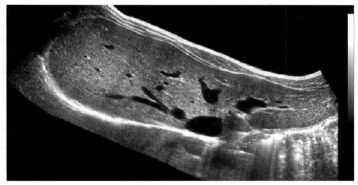

Fig. 13.4

The combination of SonoCT® scanning with tissue harmonic imaging (see p. 11) has shown promising results. It allows detailed visualization of hepatic lesions (**Fig. 13.5**) or fetal morphology in prenatal ultrasound screening (**Fig. 13.6**). The high performance computer systems now available can easily combine SieClear® or SonoCT® with three-dimensional (**Fig. 13.7**) and panoramic imaging techniques (**Fig. 13.4**). Here, almost the entire liver at the level of the hepatic venous system is visualized (see p. 36).

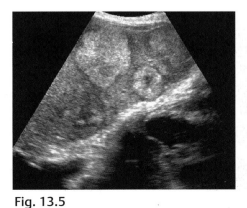

Fig. 13.5

Fig. 13.6

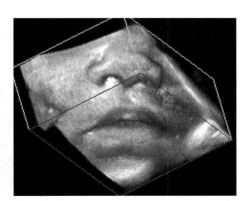

Fig. 13.7

Pulse Compression

This technique is derived from one originally developed for radar. Its main advantage is improved visualization of deep structures. It is not possible to increase penetration depth simply by increasing transmission power as this would produce undesirable thermal and mechanical effects. However, it is possible to increase the duration of the transmitted pulses and to modulate their frequency in a specific pattern ("chirp coding"). In this manner, the individual transmitted impulse has greater energy although its amplitude remains unchanged (**Fig. 14.1a**). The reflected echoes are then decoded by a chirp receiver filter and transformed back into shorter echoes of correspondingly high amplitude (**Fig. 14.1b**).

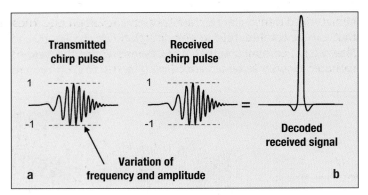

Fig. 14.1

The result is greater penetration depth with the degree of anatomic detail normally achieved only with lower frequencies and lower (and correspondingly worse) resolution. **Fig. 14.2c** shows a hypoechoic mass (**54**) deep to the thyroid gland (**81**) which would not have been visualized without pulse compression (**Fig. 14.2a**).

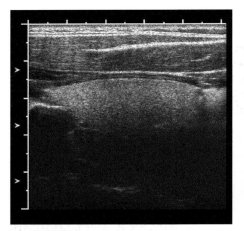

Fig. 14.2a

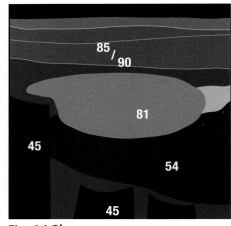

Fig. 14.2b

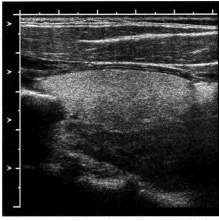

Fig. 14.2c

Precision Up-Sampling

In conventional image processing techniques with high-frequency transducers, ultrasound echoes are scanned at a rate of only about 2–5 times the speed of the maximum frequency components of the echo (wide grid in **Fig. 14.3a**). Consequently, these echoes are only detected at a few points along their curve, and the monitor image really represents only an approximation of the actual echo signal (**Fig. 14.4a**). More complex reconstruction algorithms can record the duration and amplitude of the actual echo signal far more accurately (narrower grid in **Fig. 14.3b**). The result is that the structures of a radial tendon (⬆) are visualized with significantly higher definition (**Fig. 14.4b**).

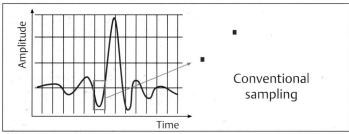

Fig. 14.3a

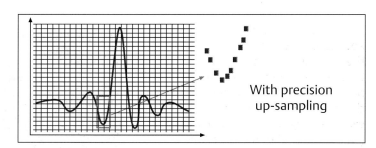

Fig. 14.3b

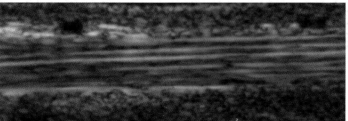

Fig. 14.4a

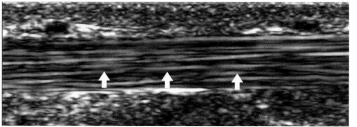

Fig. 14.4b

Diagnostic Ultrasound Catheter

Miniaturized transducers are another new development. These transducers are available in fine catheters only 3 mm in diameter that can be rotated 160° in any direction **(Fig. 15.1)**. **Fig. 15.2** shows the size of an AcuNav probe (= Accurate Navigation by Siemens) in comparison with a TEE transducer of the type used within the esophageal lumen. The small size of the disposable catheter allows it to be advanced into the heart via the venous system.

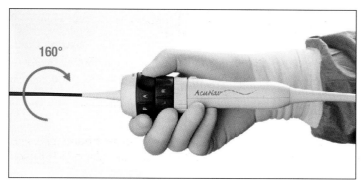

Fig. 15.1

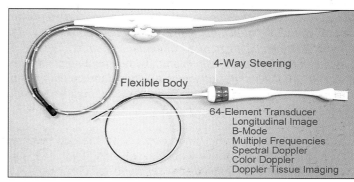

Fig. 15.2

This technique can visualize a previously poorly accessible atrial septal defect (⬇) in a B-mode scan **(Fig. 15.3a)** at higher frequencies around 7.5 MHz. It can also visualize the flow through the shunt on a color-coded Doppler image **(Fig. 15.3b)** significantly more precisely than was previously possible. This also makes it easier to monitor and verify the success of instrumental closure of the atrial septal defect (✐ in **Fig. 15.3c**). The advantages of this technique in comparison with TEE are its superior image quality and the elimination of the need for sedation or general anesthesia. This in turn makes it possible for the patient to cooperate during the examination (holding breath, Valsalva maneuver, etc.) and makes the examination less stressful for the patient.

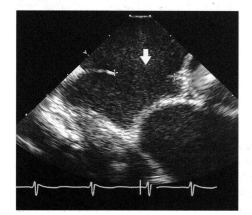

Fig. 15.3a

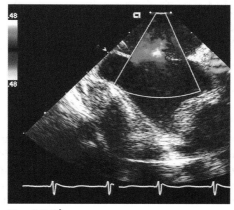

Fig. 15.3b

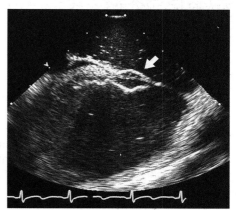

Fig. 15.3c

The catheter system can also be advanced through the right heart via the inferior vena cava and there used to guide insertion of a direct intrahepatic portosystemic shunt (DIPS). From the inferior vena cava, it is possible to visualize adjacent esophageal varices (➘ in **Fig. 15.4**) or retroperitoneal lymph nodes **(50)**, some of which are here necrotic **(109)**, with very high spatial resolution **(Fig. 15.5)**. Note that the layers of the wall (➡) of the adjacent duodenum **(80 b)** are shown in high definition.

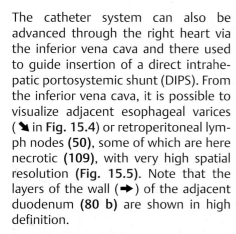

Fig. 15.4

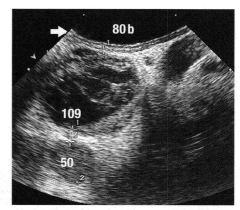

Fig. 15.5

Reverberation

The monitor image does not always reflect the true echogenicity. There are visual phenomena that do not correspond to the actual anatomy. These are referred to as "artifacts." The image generation illustrated on p. 6 assumes that the echoes always return directly from the point of reflection to the transducer. The processor makes the same assumption when computing the depth of the site of reflection. In reality, this is not always the case:

On their way back to the transducer, the reflected sound waves can encounter an impedance mismatch that reflects some of them back into deeper tissue. There they are again reflected

off an interface and reach the transducer eventually but with some delay (Fig. 16.1). The processor evaluates the delayed arrival of the returning echoes as increased penetration depth, and these echoes are visualized too far down on the image. Usually this phenomenon is lost in the background noise of the image. However, against an anechoic background such as the lumen of the urinary bladder (38) or gallbladder, these reverberations appear as lines parallel to the anterior abdominal wall (51a in Fig. 16.2). These sound waves can "bounce back and forth" repeatedly, producing a series of parallel lines (51a).

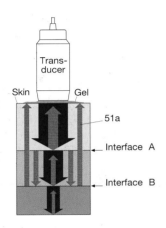

Fig. 16.1

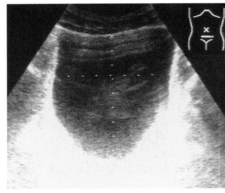

Fig. 16.2 a

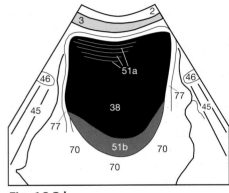

Fig. 16.2 b

Section Thickness Artifacts

The far wall of the bladder can appear similarly indistinct. If the bladder wall (77), cyst, or gallbladder is not perpendicular to the sound beam but tangential to it, the wall is indistinctly visualized and appears thickened (51b in Fig. 16.2). Such a section thickness artifact must be distinguished from layered material (small concrements, sludge, blood clots, 52 in

Fig. 16.3). However, these are usually more sharply demarcated from the remaining lumen and can be disturbed with the transducer.

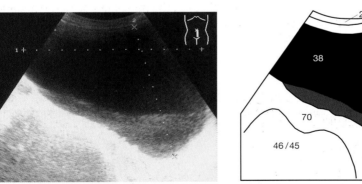

Fig. 16.3 a

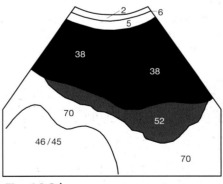

Fig. 16.3 b

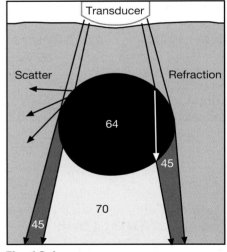

Fig. 16.4

Distal Acoustic Enhancement

Relative enhancement of the echoes (70) occurs behind large vessels or cavities (64) filled with homogeneous (anechoic) fluid (Fig. 16.4). In Figures 16.2 and 16.3 the tissue posterior to the bladder (38) appears almost white and cannot be evaluated. How does this happen?

Wherever sound waves travel for some distance through homogeneous fluid, they are not reflected and do not

attenuate. Thus there is more "unspent" acoustic energy behind the gallbladder, bladder, cysts, or major vessels than in surrounding areas of the image. This results in a more hyperechoic (brighter) appearance (70) of the underlying tissue that does not correspond to its "true" characteristics. This acoustic enhancement can also be a useful criterion for differentiating anechoic cysts (which show acoustic enhancement above a certain size) from a hypoechoic hepatic lesion (which does not usually exhibit this phenomenon).

Acoustic Shadowing

Bands of markedly reduced echogenicity (hypoechoic or anechoic = black) occur deep to strong reflectors such as ribs, concrements, some ligaments, and gastrointestinal air. As a result, the inferior ribs or the pubic bone can obscure deeper structures in the same manner as air in the stomach or bowel. The examiner can also exploit this effect to detect calcified gallstones (49) in the gallbladder (14) as in Fig. 17.1, renal calculi (49 in Fig. 56.2), or arteriosclerotic plaques (49 in Fig. 25.1). Intestinal air can either cast hypoechoic (dark) shadows or cause hyperechoic (= bright), "comet tail" artifacts due to vibration or multiple reflection.

Edge shadows (45) can occur deep to round cavities whose walls lie tangential to the sound beam (Fig. 17.2). These shadows are caused by scatter and refraction (Fig. 16.4). In the case of the gallbladder (14) in Fig. 17.2, one must examine the image carefully to

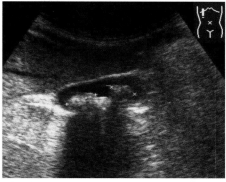

Fig. 17.1 a

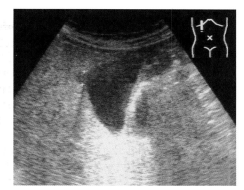

Fig. 17.2 a

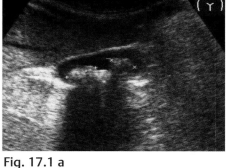

Fig. 17.1 b

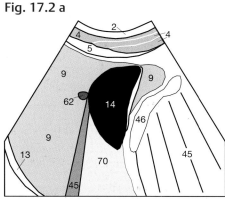

Fig. 17.2 b

correctly identify the acoustic shadow (45) as a gallbladder edge shadow and avoid mistakenly interpreting it as part of the hypoechoic less fatty portion (62) of the liver (9). Acoustic shadowing due to duodenal air (46) is commonly misinterpreted as acoustic shadows from stones in the adjacent gallbladder. Do you remember the phenomenon responsible for the false hyperechoic appearance (70) of the liver parenchyma deep to the gallbladder (14) in Fig. 17.2?

Mirror Image Artifact

Strongly reflecting interfaces such as the diaphragm (13) can deflect sound waves in such a manner that they mimic a lesion on the other side of the diaphragm (Fig. 17.3). The sound waves are deflected laterally by the diaphragm, encounter a reflector (R), and are reflected back to the diaphragm, which in turn reflects them back to the transducer. The processor can only base its calculation of the distance of the object on the time of flight of the sound pulse. Therefore, the object (R') appears too deep on the image. Fig. 17.4 shows the inferior vena cava (16) as a mirror image projected above the diaphragm (16'). Additionally, the mirror image of the hepatic parenchyma (9) appears on the pulmonary aspect of the diaphragm (9'). Fig. 37.2 shows another example of a mirror image artifact.

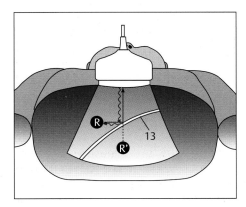

Fig. 17.3

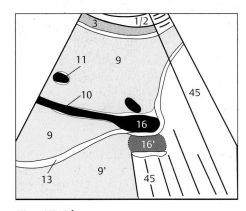

Fig. 17.4 a

Fig. 17.4 b

Side Lobe Artifact

So far, we have assumed that the sound waves propagate in a straight line from top to bottom in the image (dark blue lobe in **Fig. 18.1**). In fact, the sound waves also propagate in several secondary **"side lobes"** that can cause scatter and blurring. When such a side lobe strikes a strong reflector, the proces-sor incorrectly assigns the obliquely reflected sound waves to the adjacent lines of the image (**Fig. 18.2**). The farther later-ally the waves are reflected, the longer their path and time of flight and the deeper the processor will project the echoes on the image. This often results in an arclike extension of a strongly reflecting interface (✎ in **Fig. 18.3**).

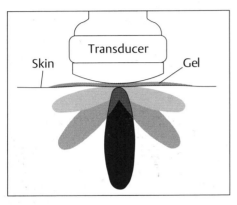

Fig. 18.1

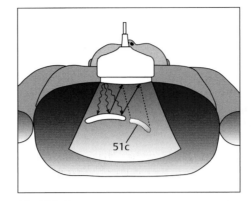

Fig. 18.2

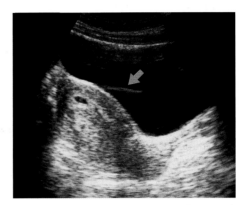

Fig. 18.3

Quiz on Technical Fundamentals and Technique

Before beginning practical exercises or Lesson 1, you are invit-ed to test which information you have really understood and are able to recall and where you still have gaps. You can check your answers by going back to the previous pages. The answer to image question 4 is on page 122.

1. Which structures are almost always anechoic (= black) on ultrasound images? Name four physiologic and four pathologic findings.

Physiologic	Pathologic
-	-
-	-
-	-
-	-

2. Which frequencies do you use for which examination and why? Specify the respective bandwidth in MHz and sketch the monitor display of the corresponding type of trans-ducer. When do you use which transducer? Why?

3. How does the processor compute the depth of the reflected echo? Can you deduce at least three artifacts from this principle and explain them to a colleague or fellow student?

4. Look at **Fig. 18.4** and explain the names and origin of all artifacts you can find.

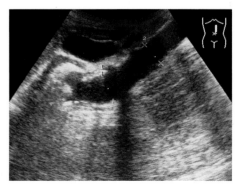

Fig. 18.4

Spatial Orientation

Before beginning practical exercises in a practice setting or an ultrasound workshop, you should first become familiar with spatial orientation in the three-dimensional space of the abdomen. To make the first step easy, we will initially consider only two perpendicular planes, the vertical (sagittal) imaging plane and the horizontal (transverse) plane. Your active participation is now required to ingrain these two planes in your memory.

Step 1: Take a (European) coffee filter (there is no hospital where you will not find one) or draw the outline of a coffee filter on a piece of paper. Most filters have the same general shape as an ultrasound image generated by a convex transducer (see p. 9).

Now imagine along which margin of the image (= edge of the coffee filter) the patient's respective anterior, posterior, left, right, cranial, and caudal structures must lie when you view the imaging plane from the patient's right side according to international convention **(Fig. 19.1a)**.

Hold the coffee filter against your abdomen and imagine that the sound waves propagate from the linea alba toward the spine. Write down four of the six possible directions on the edges of the coffee filter or your drawing. Two will be wrong, but why? (It is worth your while. You will always remember this if you figure it out for yourself.)

Step 2: Before you look up the answer, repeat the exercise for the short-axis (transverse) plane. Here, the convention is that the image is displayed on the monitor as viewed from the caudal perspective (from the patient's feet) **(Fig. 19.1b)**. Write down four of the six possible directions on the back of the filter. Again two will be wrong, but different ones this time. Once you have thought about your results, check the answer on page 122.

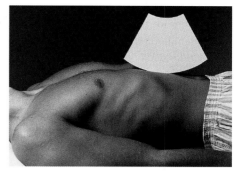

Fig. 19.1 a

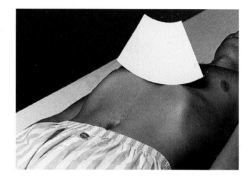

Fig. 19.1 b

The next problem will be the acoustic shadow created by superimposed intestinal air. The solution is usually <u>not</u> to use more gel (as many beginners think) but to vary the pressure applied to the transducer.

How Much Pressure Should I Apply to the Transducer?

The beginner is usually concerned about causing discomfort to the patient and does not press the transducer firmly against the abdominal wall. As a result of this hesitation (↓↓↓), the air normally present in the lumen of the stomach or bowel **(26)** remains in place and its acoustic shadow **(45)** obscures the view of the pancreas **(33)** and adjacent vessels posterior to it **(Fig. 19.2a)**. The extrahepatic common bile duct **(66)** and portal vein **(11)** are also often obscured by gastric or duodenal air.

The solution in adults is to apply measured, slowly increasing pressure (**↓↓↓**). Do not apply pressure too suddenly so as

not to startle the patient or cause unnecessary pain (**Fig. 19.3**). The trick is to maintain this pressure. That will increasingly and gently displace intestinal air from the imaging plane. The acoustic shadow will disappear after some seconds and the pancreas **(33)** and other vessels will be clearly visualized **(Fig. 19.2b)**.

This principle is especially helpful for visualizing retroperitoneal lymph nodes and vessels even in the mid and lower abdomen. In infants, this maneuver is usually superfluous and counterproductive because of their lower pain threshold and defensive reaction.

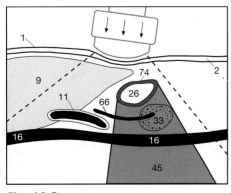

Fig. 19.2 a

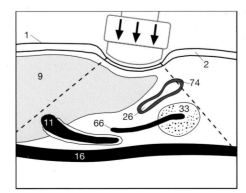

Fig. 19.2 b

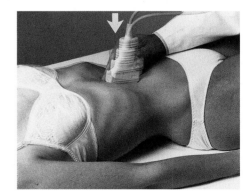

Fig. 19.3

Relevance of Adequate Breathing Instructions

Beginners are naturally reluctant to give the patient very direct instructions. Nonetheless, almost all patients are very cooperative when you explain the following situation to them: Image quality (and therefore the validity of your findings) in the upper abdomen is often markedly improved when the patient inhales very deeply to displace the liver caudally. Why?

In a neutral breathing position (**Fig. 20.1a**), the liver and spleen are not the only structures obscured by acoustic shadows of the caudal lung segments. Often the pancreas (**33**) and its surroundings cannot be visualized because of the air content of the stomach (**26**). However, when the liver is displaced caudally (→) in maximum inspiration (**Fig. 20.1b**), the air-filled stomach (**26**) and bowel are also displaced caudally, allowing a good view of the pancreas and important lymph nodes. The same principle greatly improves visualization of the kidneys and hilum of the liver, which move with respiration (see below).

Please use clear breathing instructions such as: "Take a deep breath with your mouth open [pause] and now please hold your breath." Remember to instruct the patient immediately to exhale after an adequate pause (maximum of 20 seconds) or as soon as you have frozen the image. This instruction is not nearly as trivial as you may think.

Good breathing instructions are not only well received by the patient, they also avoid undue strain on the patient's respiratory system and expedite the examination of the upper abdomen. These maneuvers are superfluous when examining the lower abdomen.

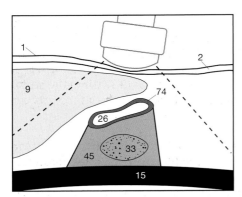

Fig. 20.1a

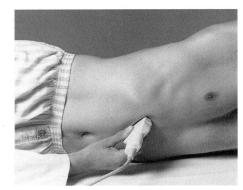

Fig. 20.1b

Visualizing the Hilum of the Liver

Should you be unable to visualize the hilum of the liver despite the tricks discussed above, try to visualize the porta hepatis through an intercostal window in expiration (**Fig. 20.2**). If this is also unsuccessful, place the patient in the left lateral decubitus position (**Fig. 20.3**). The liver's own weight will shift it closer to the anterior abdominal wall, displacing bowel loops and exposing the porta hepatis with its important vascular structures (see p. 32).

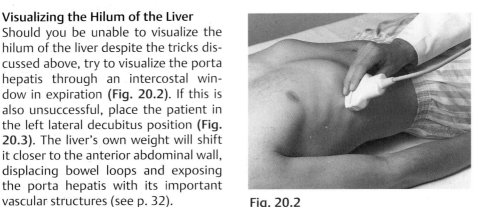

Fig. 20.2   **Fig. 20.3**

Test Your Skills:

Please look at **Fig. 20.4** and **20.5**. Both show poor quality images. Determine which was obtained with too little gel and which with too little pressure. **Fig. 20.6** shows an optimal image obtained with proper pressure and an adequate amount of gel. All three images were obtained in the same patient in rapid succession. The answer is on page 122.

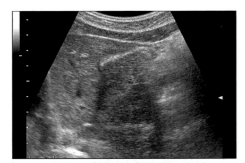

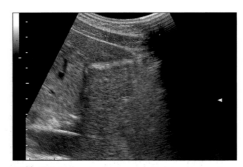

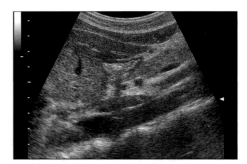

Fig. 20.4   **Fig. 20.5**   **Fig. 20.6**

Before you work through this page, please complete the exercise on page 19 to familiarize yourself with spatial orientation in sagittal planes. You should only proceed here when you are completely familiar with this orientation and the physical principles discussed on pp. 6–18. From here on, you will be assumed to have this basic knowledge.

The **goal** of examining the retroperitoneum goes beyond evaluation of the retroperitoneal vessels. It is also intended to exclude disorders such as aortic aneurysm or thrombosis of the inferior vena cava. An additional goal is to become familiar with the vascular anatomy of this region because obliquely imaged vessels can easily be mistaken for oval lymph nodes, which are also hypoechoic. Correct identification of the individual vessels also greatly facilitates spatial orientation and provides landmarks to aid in identifying other structures later.

The **transducer** is placed on the epigastrium along the linea alba perpendicular to the abdominal wall, and the beam is swept through the upper abdomen in a fanlike motion (**Fig. 21.1**). For now, commit only the normal cross-sectional anatomy to memory: When you tilt the

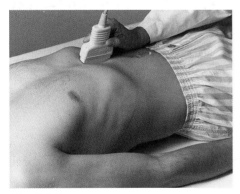

Fig. 21.1

transducer to the patient's right side (**Fig. 21.2a**), you will find the aorta (**15**), the celiac trunk (**32**), and the superior mesenteric artery (SMA, **17**) posterior to the liver (**9**) and anterior to the vertebra. At the left margin of the image you will see the thin hyperechoic line of the diaphragm (bare area, **13**) that exhibits a hypoechoic muscular extension (**13a**) at the anterior margin of the aorta, which like the esophagus (**34**) can easily be mistaken for a retroperitoneal lymph node. Farther inferiorly, the left renal vein (**25**) is shown in transverse section as it crosses between the superior mesenteric artery (**17**) and the aorta (**15**). Beginners often misinterpret the hypoechoic oval shape of this vein as a pathologic lymph node. Compare this to the cross section at the same level (**Fig. 28.3**) and the anatomic sketch in **Fig. 27.2**. Farther anteriorly (closer to the transducer) you will find the confluence of the portal vein (**12**) at the posterior margin of the pancreas (**33**). Air in the stomach (**26**) can produce acoustic shadows at the inferior margin of the liver.

Now tilt the transducer to the patient's left side (**Fig. 21.3a**) to visualize the inferior vena cava (IVC, **16**) in a right paravertebral location and its junction with the right atrium (**116**). The diameter of the aorta and inferior vena cava are measured perpendicular to their longitudinal axes (see pp. 23–25). Hepatic veins (**10**), branches of the left portal venous branch (**11**) and, anterior to it, the hepatic artery (**18**) can be identified within the liver (**9**). A thin hyperechoic septum at this level separates the caudate lobe (**9a**) from the rest of the hepatic parenchyma (**9**). The maximum craniocaudal diameter of the caudate lobe should measure less than 5.0 cm and its anteroposterior diameter less than 2.5 cm.

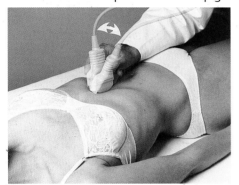

Fig. 21.2 a

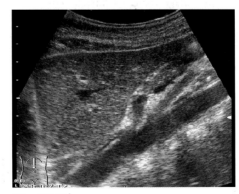

Fig. 21.2 b

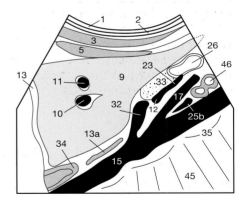

Fig. 21.2 c

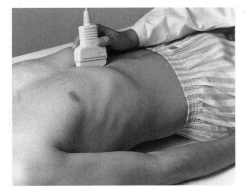

Fig. 21.3 a

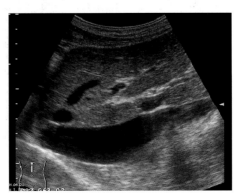

Fig. 21.3 b

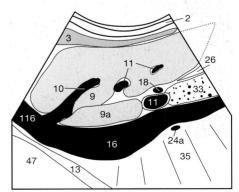

Fig. 21.3 c

After you have examined the upper retroperitoneum, move the transducer inferiorly (➡) along the aorta and inferior vena cava (**Fig. 22.1a**). In addition to visualizing the lumens of these major vessels, the examiner must also tilt the transducer (**Fig. 21.1**) to search for enlarged perivascular lymph nodes on either side of the vessels. Enlarged lymph nodes will invariably appear as hypoechoic oval structures (see pp. 24 and 31). Abnormally enlarged lymph nodes can also occur anterior and posterior to the major vessels and in the aortocaval space. In the absence of a retro-aortic mass, the distance between the posterior wall of the aorta and the anterior margins of the vertebrae should not exceed 5 mm. It is always best to perform this examination in two planes (see pp. 27 and 28).

The iliac vessels arising caudal to the aortic bifurcation are identified in the same manner and examined in two planes, parallel to the axis of the vessel (**Fig. 22.1b**) and perpendicular to it (**Fig. 22.1c**).

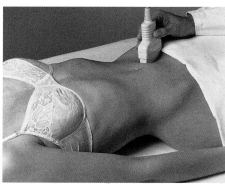

Fig. 22.1 a

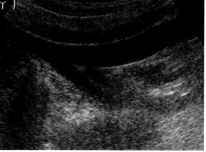

Fig. 22.1 b

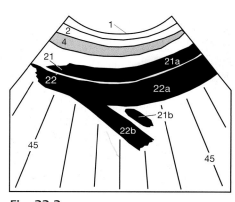

Fig. 22.1 c

The confluence of the external iliac vein (**22a**) and internal iliac vein (**22b**) is a common site for enlarged regional lymph nodes (**Fig. 22.2**). The iliac artery (**21**) is anterior to the vein (above it on the image). When in doubt, a simple compression test can help you distinguish the two vessels. Because of its lower intraluminal pressure, the vein is more easily compressed with the transducer than the artery.

On the transverse image (**Fig. 22.3**), one can often distinguish iliac vessels from hypoechoic bowel contents in loops of the small bowel (**46**) by intestinal peristalsis alone. If necessary, one can try to induce peristalsis by rapidly varying the pressure applied to the transducer.

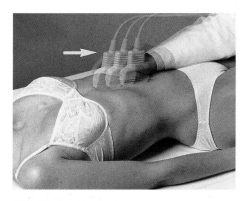

Fig. 22.2 a

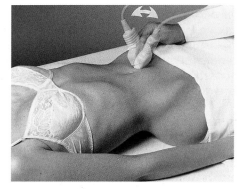

Fig. 22.2 b

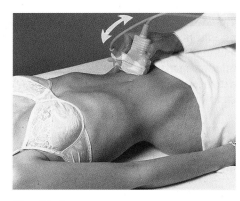

Fig. 22.2 c

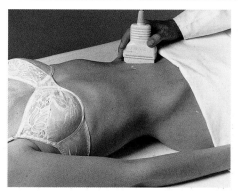

Fig. 22.3 a

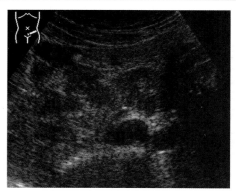

Fig. 22.3 b

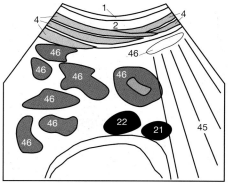

Fig. 22.3 c

Circumscribed dilations of the vascular lumen usually occur as a result of arteriosclerotic lesions and localized weakening of the arterial wall, and, less often, secondary to trauma. Ectasia is defined as a dilation of the aortic lumen greater than 25 mm and less than 30 mm. It can also occur in combination with an aneurysm (Fig. 23.1), which is defined as a diameter greater than 30 mm in the suprarenal abdominal aorta or 40 mm in the aortic arch.

The dilation can be fusiform or saccular. Complications can include dissection of the layers of the aortic wall (dissecting aneurysm) or mural thrombosis (52), which can lead to peripheral or abdominal emboli. Risk factors for rupture include increasing aneurysm size, diameter exceeding 50 or 60 mm, respectively, and outpouching of the wall resembling a diverticulum. A concentric lumen in a thrombosed aneurysm can have a protective effect, whereas an eccentric lumen is deemed to be at increased risk of rupture. As a rule, the risk of rupture increases with aneurysm size. However, the indication for surgical intervention depends on many individual factors so that it is not possible to define an absolute threshold.

Any ultrasound evaluation of an aneurysm must determine the following crucial facts: The maximum craniocaudal length of the dilation (Fig. 23.2), its maximum transverse diameter (Fig. 23.3), and any dissections, thrombosis, and involvement of visceral branch arteries (celiac trunk, superior mesenteric artery, renal arteries, and iliac arteries).

The primary artery supplying the spinal cord (great radicular artery of Adamkiewicz) is variable in its segmental level, and because of its narrow caliber it is not usually detected on ultrasound images. Supplementary spiral CT or angiography are usually required to visualize the arterial supply to the spinal cord.

Checklist for Aortic Aneurysm

Suprarenal aorta < 25 mm (normal)
Aortic ectasia: 25–30 mm
Aneurysm: > 30 mm
Signs of increased rupture risk:

- Progressive dilation
- Diameter > 60 mm
- Saccular not fusiform
- Evidence of dissection
- Eccentric lumen

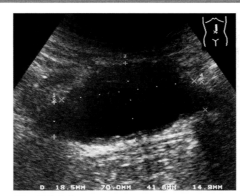

Fig. 23.1 a

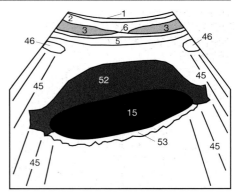

Fig. 23.1 b

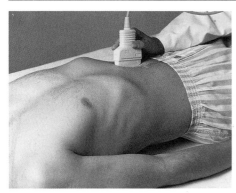

Fig. 23.2 a

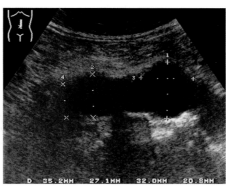

Fig. 23.2 b

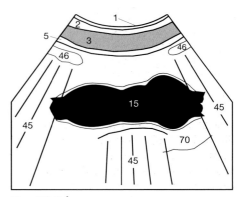

Fig. 23.2 c

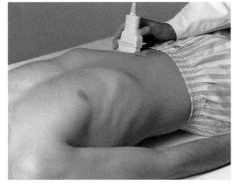

Fig. 23.3 a

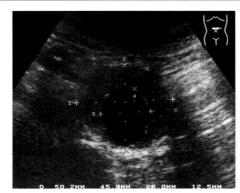

Fig. 23.3 b

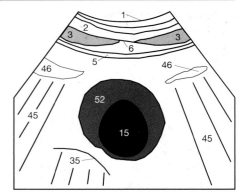

Fig. 23.3 c

Lymph nodes **(55)** normally appear as hypoechoic oval structures. It is important to distinguish them from vascular structures visualized end on or obliquely, which can exhibit the same characteristics on static images. Therefore, our ultrasound courses train the student to continuously sweep the transducer through an arc to visualize each region dynamically in two planes. Using this technique, one will find that blood vessels either widen (and join other vessels) or taper, whereas lymph nodes appear and disappear abruptly. Examiners who simply move the transducer back and forth at random fail to exploit this distinguishing characteristic.

In the lower abdomen, small bowel loops with hypoechoic content visualized end on can mimic lymph nodes in the absence of peristalsis. A differential diagnosis must also consider thrombosed veins. Causes of lymph node enlargement other than reactive inflammation or metastases of malignant processes include lymphomatous infiltration in Hodgkin disease or non-Hodgkin lymphoma.

Diagnostic Classification of Enlarged Lymph Nodes

Depending on its location, a normal abdominal lymph node is reported to measure 7–10 mm along its long axis. Physiologically larger lymph nodes measuring up to 20 mm **(Fig. 24.3)** occur along the external iliac arteries and in the inguinal region. Normal and reactive inflammatory lymph nodes are typically oval, and the ratio of the long axis to the short axis is greater than 2:1. This means that a lymph node is over twice as long as it is wide with the transducer held parallel to the long axis.

The "hilum sign" or "hilum fat sign" in which the hyperechoic hilar architecture of an enlarged lymph node is surrounded by a hypoechoic periphery, also suggests a benign process. Such lymph nodes are often encountered in the setting of hepatitis, pancreatitis **(Fig. 29.3)**, cholecystitis, or cholangitis at the porta hepatis **(Fig. 33.3)**.

Spherical lymph nodes (in which the ratio of the long axis to the short axis is about 1:1) without a hilum sign suggest a pathologic change. A lymph node infiltrated by lymphoma is usually more markedly hypoechoic than an inflamed or metastatic lymph node. The perfusion pattern of a lymph node on color duplex sonography can provide additional information (see pp. 104–106 and *Teaching Manual of Color Duplex Sonography* on page 127).

Wherever enlarged lymph nodes are encountered, follow-up examinations are important to check for progressive enlargement, central liquefaction (an abscess produces an anechoic center), or regression such as can occur after chemotherapy of the underlying disorder. Liver and spleen size should also be measured and documented in lymphoma patients.

The location of the primary tumor can be inferred from the known lymphatic pathway; a testicular tumor should be excluded in young men with enlarged para-aortic lymph nodes at the level of the renal arteries.

Malignant lymphomas may press upon or displace adjacent vascular structures **(Fig. 24.2)** but they usually neither invade their walls nor infiltrate other adjacent organs (see p. 31). Non-Hodgkin lymphoma often involves the mesenteric lymph nodes **(55)** **(Figs. 24.1 and 24.2)**, whereas Hodgkin disease shows a predilection for thoracic and retroperitoneal lymph nodes.

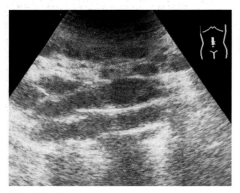

Fig. 24.1 a

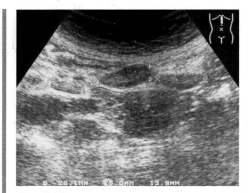

Fig. 24.2 a

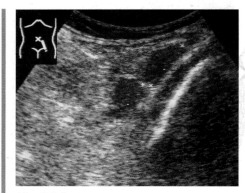

Fig. 24.3 a

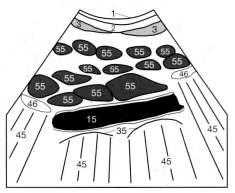

Fig. 24.1 b

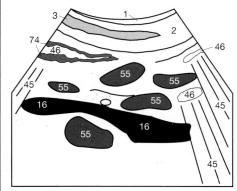

Fig. 24.2 b

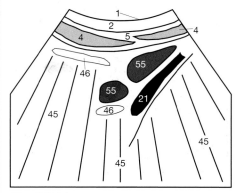

Fig. 24.3 b

Systematic examination of the retroperitoneum must include evaluation of the venous system in addition to any changes in the aorta and lymph nodes. The inferior vena cava (IVC) can be distinguished from the aorta by its anatomic location (right prevertebral location, not left). A further distinguishing characteristic is its typical precordial double pulse (as opposed to the single pulse of the aorta). Older patients often exhibit echogenic arteriosclerotic plaques (49) along the wall of the aorta (15, Fig. 25.1). When calcified, these lesions can create acoustic shadows (45).

Right Heart Failure

When evaluating the inferior vena cava (16), be alert to any dilation exceeding 20 mm (25 mm in young athletes) as this suggests venous congestion proximal to the right atrium consistent with right heart failure (Fig. 25.2). It is important to obtain the measurements perpendicular to the longitudinal axis of the vein. Be careful to avoid exaggerating the size of the lumen of the vena cava by mistakenly including hepatic veins (10) that enter the vena cava inferior to the diaphragm (Fig. 25.2). When in doubt, perform the vena cava collapse test during forced inspiration. Instruct the patient to inhale as deeply as possible through the nose with the mouth closed. The sudden drop in intrapleural pressure collapses the subdiaphragmatic vena cava or at least briefly reduces its diameter to one-third or less of its initial value.

The challenge for the examiner is to maintain the imaging plane in the center of the inferior vena cava during the sudden expansion of the chest on inspiration. Alternatively, this test can be performed when imaging the upper abdomen in the transverse plane, or the diameter of the peripheral hepatic veins may be evaluated (see p. 36).

Do you remember the reason why the liver tissue in Fig. 25.2 posterior to the distended inferior vena cava appears to be more hyperechoic than anterior to it? If not, please review the artifacts on page 9 and name this phenomenon.

Images of the distal iliac vessels (Fig. 25.3) can occasionally show a hematoma (50) in the vicinity of the iliac artery (21) or vein (22) secondary to an inguinal puncture. Persistent blood flow into the hematoma through a patent communication with the arterial lumen is referred to as a "false aneurysm." This is distinguished from a true aneurysm by the fact that there is no outpouching of all layers of the vascular wall but a perivascular hematoma secondary to a full thickness tear in the wall (Fig. 25.3). A differential diagnosis must distinguish subacute or acute inguinal hernias from psoas major abscesses within the true pelvis, lymphoceles, synovial cysts in the hip and larger ovarian cysts, and from metastases with central liquefactive necrosis (57).

Checklist for Right Heart Failure

- IVC dilated   > 20 mm or
                 > 25 mm in young athletes

- Dilated hepatic veins > 6 mm
  in the periphery of the liver
- IVC does not collapse on forced inspiration
- Possible pleural effusion,
  often initially unilateral on the right

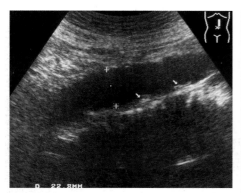

Fig. 25.1 a

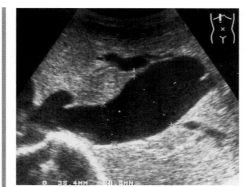

Fig. 25.2 a

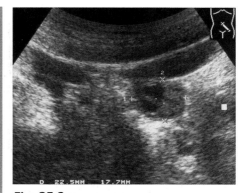

Fig. 25.3 a

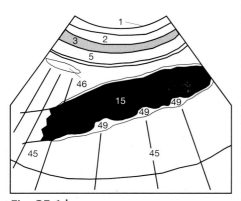

Fig. 25.1 b

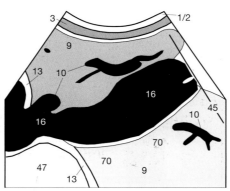

Fig. 25.2 b

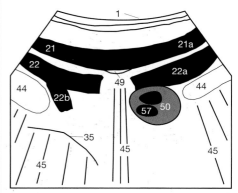

Fig. 25.3 b

Before proceeding to the material in Lesson 2, you can test whether you have really mastered the learning points and contents of Lesson 1 by answering the questions below. Pursued with a little determination, this self evaluation can effectively prevent you from simply skimming through this workbook superficially without any long-term benefit from your reading.

1. Which anatomic direction corresponds to the left edge of the image on sagittal scans? For practice, label the coffee filter shown here. Remember which of the following six anatomic directions cannot appear on the edges of the filter: anterior, posterior, left, right, cranial, caudal.

2. What is the maximum normal luminal diameter of the inferior vena cava and abdominal aorta? What is the definition of aortic ectasia and aortic aneurysm? What questions would you as an examiner seek to answer using ultrasound images? What are the limits of ultrasound imaging (when would supplementary CT or DSA be better)?

3. Which five physiologic structures can mimic hypoechoic lymph nodes on a sagittal image of the upper abdominal aorta? Please specify all five and draw their position in the standard imaging plane from memory.

4. Which two supplementary ultrasound examinations do you perform to quickly exclude or confirm right heart failure suggested by a borderline diameter of the inferior vena cava and suspicious clinical signs (without ECG)?

5. What is the maximum length of the long axis of retroperitoneal lymph nodes that may still be regarded as physiologic? Name the diagnostic criteria for classifying lymph nodes and their respective normal values. What is the value of follow-up examinations in the presence of abnormally enlarged lymph nodes?

6. Look at the three transducers shown here **(Fig. 26.1)**. Please write each one's name above it and its frequency ranges and areas of application below it. Can you give reasons for your answers?

Enjoy the test.
You will find the answers to questions 1 through 6 on the preceding pages. You may look up the answers to the image in question 7 on page 123 (but of course only after working through the individual questions).

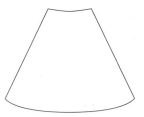

Suprarenal aorta <	mm	Infrarenal aorta <	mm
IVC (in athlete) <	mm	Aortic ectasia ~	mm
Aortic aneurysm >	mm		

a) _____

b) _____

c) _____

d) _____

e) _____

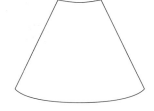

a) _____

b) _____

7. Evaluate this quiz image step by step **(Fig. 26.2)**. Which imaging plane is shown here? Which organs and/or vessels are visualized? Try to name all the structures in the image. How does this image differ from normal findings? Please provide a differential diagnosis.

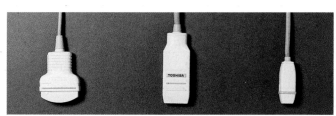

Fig. 26.1

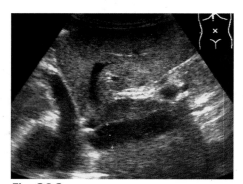

Fig. 26.2

Before you work through the next few pages, you should again review the transverse imaging planes: Where is the liver (on the patient's right side) visualized on a correctly oriented transverse scan? On the right or left side of the image? If you are not completely sure of the answer, please go back to page 19 and review the relative anatomic location of the organs in the transverse planes with the aid of the coffee filter (the solution is found on page 122).

In addition to evaluation of the pancreas, the goals of this examination include evaluation of the perivascular lymph node groups. To image the transverse planes of the upper abdomen, rotate the transducer 90° counterclockwise and place it horizontally on the upper abdomen. The patient is instructed to inhale deeply, and the upper abdomen is systematically scanned

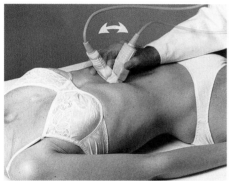

by sweeping the transducer slowly and steadily through a craniocaudal arc (**Fig. 27.1**). In this manner, vessels can be easily evaluated over their entire length and differentiated from focal masses.

Fig. 27.1

The problem for the examiner is that these imaging planes show numerous arteries, veins, bile ducts, and lymph nodes in close proximity to each other, all of which must be differentiated from each other despite similar echogenicity (blood vessels are anechoic to hypoechoic, as are lymph nodes).

Do you remember where the left renal vein crosses to the contralateral right side and whether the right renal artery courses anterior or posterior to the inferior vena cava on its way to the right kidney? Refresh your knowledge of basic anatomy by labeling all the numbered structures in **Fig. 27.2** in the blanks below the figure, initially without consulting the legend or an anatomy book. This approach may appear somewhat cumbersome at first, but your retention will be significantly better than if you were to simply reproduce a labeled drawing. Next, compare your answers to the legend on the back cover flap and make any necessary corrections. Please repeat this exercise with a little determination on separate sheets of paper until you are able to label every numbered structure in **Figs. 27.2** and **27.3** correctly. Only then should you proceed to the following pages, as both the concept of this workbook and the structure of our practical ultrasound courses absolutely require this knowledge.

Fig. 27.3 illustrates once again the topographic relationship of the pancreas, duodenum, and spleen to the major upper abdominal blood vessels. To help consolidate this knowledge, the three most important standard transverse imaging planes of the upper abdomen are shown on the next page.

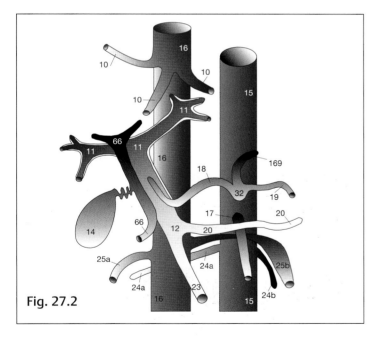

Fig. 27.2

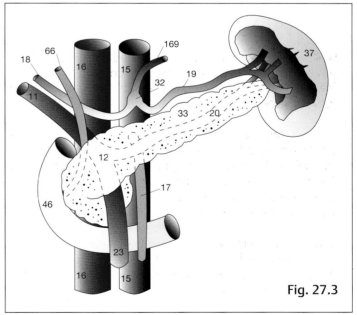

Fig. 27.3

Please complete the list with the aid of both figures. Which number corresponds to which anatomic structure?

10 = _____

11 = _____

12 = _____

14 = _____

15 = _____

16 = _____

17 = _____

18 = _____

19 = _____

20 = _____

23 = _____

24 a = _____

24 b = _____

25a = _____

25b = _____

32 = _____

33 = _____

37 = _____

46 = _____

66 = _____

169 = _____

Usually you begin by instructing the patient to take a deep breath and hold it so as to shift the liver caudally and create a better acoustic window for imaging the pancreas, lesser sac, and origins of the major vessels (see p. 20).

The hyperechoic skin (1), the hypoechoic subcutaneous fatty tissue (2), and the two rectus abdominis muscles (3) are directly beneath the transducer. The cranial transverse plane (**Fig. 28.1**) visualizes the celiac trunk (32) with two of its branches, the hepatic artery (18) and splenic artery (19). Their configuration often resembles the fluke of a whale. Posterior to the linea alba (6) and farther caudally (**Figs. 28.2** and **28.3**) lies the rhomboid extension of the ligamentum teres (7) and the obliterated umbilical vein. The lesser sac appears as a narrow cleft posterior to the liver (9); the pancreas (33) lies immediately posterior to it. The tail of the pancreas is often obscured by acoustic shadows (45) from gas in the stomach (26). The

splenic vein (20) invariably courses directly along the posterior aspect of the pancreas. The left renal vein (25) lies farther posterior between the superior mesenteric artery (SMA, 17) and the aorta (15), but farther caudal (**Fig. 28.3**). Between these two planes, the superior mesenteric artery (17) arises from the aorta (15). Here one will occasionally find an atypical origin of the hepatic artery arising from the superior mesenteric artery. The origins of the celiac trunk and superior mesenteric artery often lie immediately beneath one another; please check this on the sagittal section as well (**Fig. 21.2**).

Note that this projection inverts the position of all the organs and vessels. The teardrop-shaped inferior vena cava (16) is on the left side of the image, the round aorta (15) on the right anterior to the anterior margin of the vertebra (35). The head of the pancreas typically surrounds the confluence (12) of the portal vein (11), which is often obscured by duodenal air (46) at the porta hepatis.

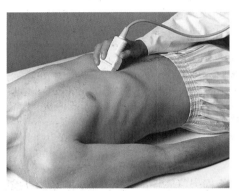

Fig. 28.1 a

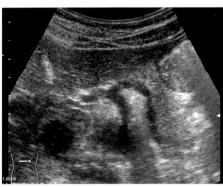

Fig. 28.1 b

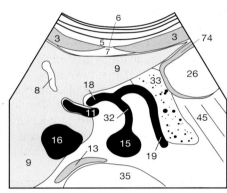

Fig. 28.1 c

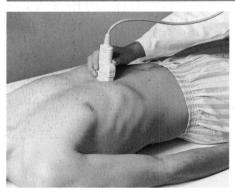

Fig. 28.2 a

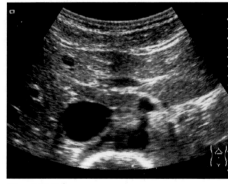

Fig. 28.2 b

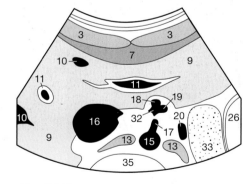

Fig. 28.2 c

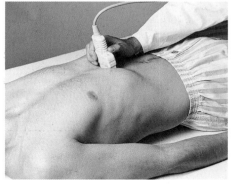

Fig. 28.3 a

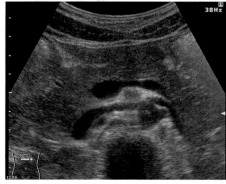

Fig. 28.3 b

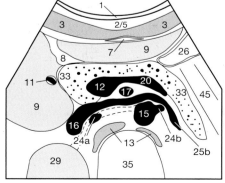

Fig. 28.3 c

Age-related Echogenicity

The echogenicity of the pancreatic parenchyma changes with increasing age. In young and slender patients, it is hypoechoic like their hepatic parenchyma (Fig. 28.3b). In obese patients or with increasing age (Fig. 30.1a), the impedance mismatches intensify in the increasingly heterogeneous pancreatic parenchyma and the pancreas becomes more hyperechoic (brighter).

The normal maximum anteroposterior diameter of the pancreas is somewhat variable; in the head it is < 3 cm, in the body < 2 cm, and in the tail < 2.5 cm.

Common causes of pancreatitis include impaired drainage of secretion due to a gallstones lodged in the distal common bile duct (biliary pancreatitis), increased viscosity of the pancreatic secretion in parenteral nutrition, and alcoholic pancreatitis, which is thought to result in part from obstruction of the small pancreatic ducts by protein precipitates.

Acute Pancreatitis

First-degree acute pancreatitis can initially occur without any ultrasound imaging correlate. However, extensive inflammation is accompanied by a markedly hypoechoic edema, and the pancreas (33) may be poorly demarcated from its surroundings. The real value of ultrasound is not in making the initial diagnosis of pancreatitis. This is done more reliably by enzymatic serum tests and computed tomography, especially as ultrasound evaluation in the acute stage is rendered very difficult by the pain and the presence of gas.

Chronic Pancreatitis

Chronic pancreatitis on the other hand is characterized by inhomogeneous fibrosis of the pancreas (Fig. 29.1) with areas of nodular calcification (53) and an undulating, irregular contour of the organ (Figs. 29.1 and 29.2). The pancreatic duct (75) can also exhibit an irregular luminal diameter resembling a string of pearls (Fig. 29.2). The normal duct is smoothly demarcated with a luminal diameter of 1–2 mm. Reactive inflammatory enlargement of lymph nodes (55) may occur in the vicinity of the pancreas (Fig. 29.3), for instance, anterior to the portal vein (11).

Ultrasound is important in excluding other disease entities in a differential diagnosis (such as cholecystitis, choledocholithiasis, or aortic aneurysm), in evaluating the course of the disease, and in excluding complications secondary to pancreatitis. These include thrombosis of the splenic vein (20), which can require supplementary color duplex sonography. Ultrasound can also visualize inflammatory infiltration of the adjacent duodenal or gastric wall (46, 26) and pseudocysts. Prompt detection of retroperitoneal lines of necrosis (grade II acute pancreatitis) is also important to allow surgical intervention or ultrasound or CT-guided aspiration.

The inflammation does not always involve the entire pancreas. Segmental or "groove" pancreatitis confined to individual sections of the gland has also been observed. It is often difficult to distinguish these forms of pancreatitis from other focal masses such as a carcinoma.

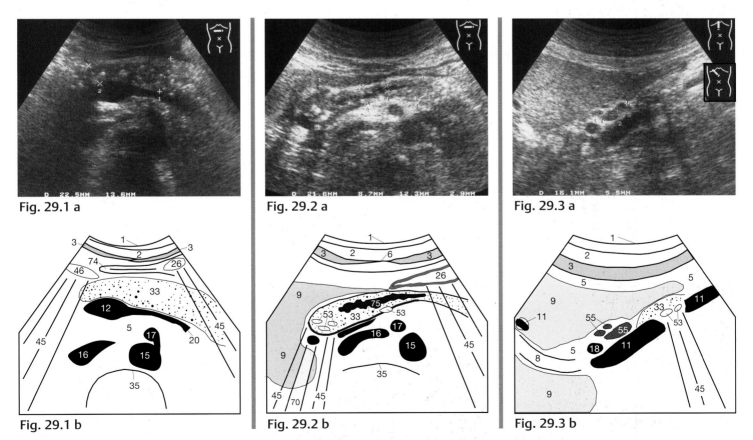

Fig. 29.1 a   Fig. 29.2 a   Fig. 29.3 a

Fig. 29.1 b   Fig. 29.2 b   Fig. 29.3 b

The normal echogenicity of the pancreas (33) in **Fig. 21.2** or **Fig. 28.3** does not differ appreciably from the echogenicity of the hepatic parenchyma. Increasing age or obesity leads to a uniform increase in echogenicity that is referred to as pancreatic lipomatosis (**Fig. 30.1**). This greatly increases the contrast to the anechoic splenic vein (20) and the confluence of the portal vein (12).

Pancreatic tumors (54) are often more hypoechoic than the rest of the parenchyma and are difficult to distinguish from adjacent bowel loops (check for peristalsis) or peripancreatic lymph nodes (**Fig. 30.2**). Pancreatic carcinomas generally have a poor prognosis. Depending on their location, they often remain clinically silent for a long time and are often detected late. They are often identified in diagnostic examinations seeking the cause of compression of the distal common bile duct with resultant cholestasis or unexplained weight loss.

Early retroperitoneal extension, nodal or hepatic metastases, and / or peritoneal carcinomatosis are responsible for the poor five-year survival rate, which is less than 10%.

Because of their peripheral hormonal effect, endocrine pancreatic tumors are often smaller when diagnosed. Like all small pancreatic processes, they are better visualized on endoscopic ultrasound (**Fig. 30.3**). An annular transducer on the tip of an endoscope is advanced into the stomach or duodenum. The transducer is surrounded by a water-filled balloon to facilitate acoustic coupling with the gastric or duodenal wall.

Because of the close proximity of the target organ, higher frequencies (5.0–10.0 MHz) can be used to achieve higher spatial resolution.

Bear in mind that the tail of the pancreas can be better visualized by slightly rotating the transducer counterclockwise out of the transverse plane (**Fig. 30.4**).

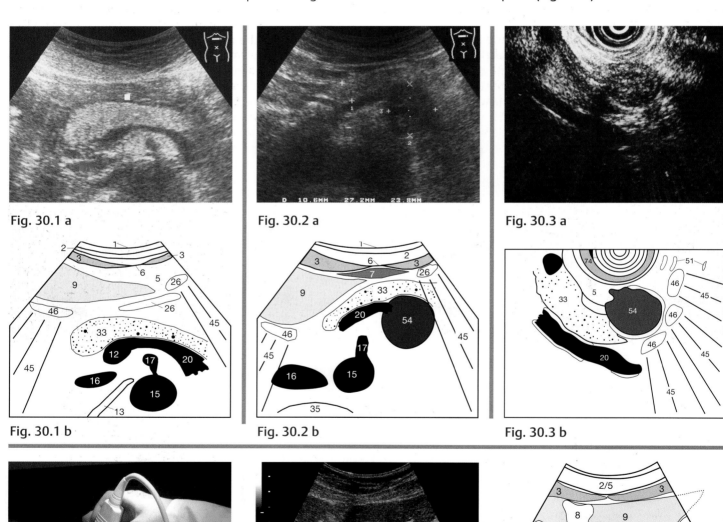

Fig. 30.1 a

Fig. 30.2 a

Fig. 30.3 a

Fig. 30.1 b

Fig. 30.2 b

Fig. 30.3 b

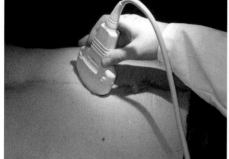

Fig. 30.4 a

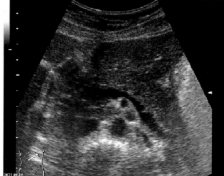

Fig. 30.4 b

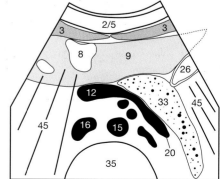

Fig. 30.4 c

Do you remember the criteria for distinguishing inflammatory enlarged lymph nodes from lymphomatous lymph nodes and nodal metastases of other primary tumors? If not, please go back to page 24 or see pages 104–106 and review the differential diagnostic possibilities discussed there.

Especially under conditions not conducive to ultrasound examination (such as in very obese patients), it is important to reliably distinguish physiologic vessels imaged end on or obliquely (**15, 16**) from pathologic lymph nodes (**55**) (**Figs. 31.1** and **31.2**). Precise knowledge of normal vascular anatomy is crucial. Markedly hypoechoic lymph nodes lacking a hyperechoic hilum that displace but do not invade adjacent veins suggest lymphoma such as in chronic lymphatic leukemia (if this repetition bores you, then you have already mastered one of the learning points ...).

Fig. 31.2 shows a pathologic lymph node directly to the right of and anterior to the bifurcation of the celiac trunk (**32**) into the common hepatic artery (**18**) and splenic artery (**19**). The mass effect of the lymph node has caused the celiac trunk to lose its typical shape resembling the fluke of a diving whale. In **Fig. 31.1** a lymph node conglomerate (**55**) has displaced the hepatic artery (**18**) so far anteriorly that the segment near the celiac trunk exhibits an atypically elongated and straight course.

Lymph node conglomerates can occasionally encase retroperitoneal or mesenteric vessels. In such cases, readily identifiable lymph nodes are measured and documented on the image so that follow-up studies can determine the extent of growth in the interim.

One rule of thumb to remember is to measure the size of the liver and spleen whenever enlarged intra-abdominal or retroperitoneal lymph nodes are encountered. Both organs should then be carefully examined for inhomogeneous infiltrations. Harmonic imaging techniques in combination with contrast agents (see p. 12) can be helpful in such cases (**Fig. 12.7**).

Without these methods, diffuse lymphomatous infiltration of the spleen will not necessarily produce detectable morphologic changes in the splenic parenchyma. An infiltrated spleen can appear normal or may only show diffuse enlargement on noncontrasted ultrasound images (**Fig. 72.1**).

The cervical, axillary, and inguinal nodes must also be examined for possible enlargement. Rarely, paralytic fluid-filled bowel loops can be mistaken for mesenteric lymph nodes. A bowel diverticulum (**54**) can also mimic a tumor or an enlarged lymph node (**Fig 31.3**). Occasionally, the differential diagnosis can be clarified by alternately applying and relieving compression with the transducer to provoke peristaltic activity in a paralytic bowel loop.

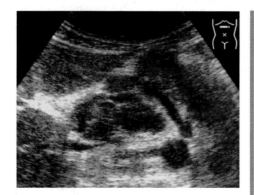

Fig. 31.1 a

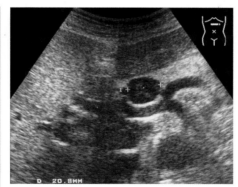

Fig. 31.2 a

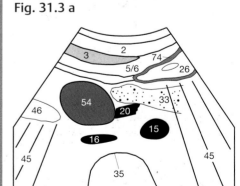

Fig. 31.3 a

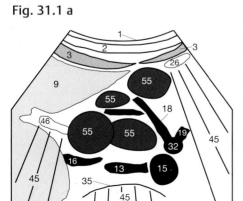

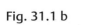
Fig. 31.1 b

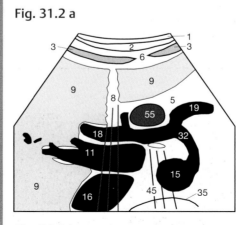

Fig. 31.2 b

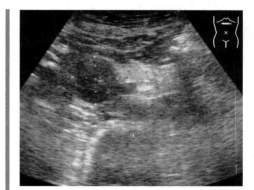

Fig. 31.3 b

To obtain the standard plane for the porta hepatis, the transducer is rotated a few degrees clockwise (Fig. 32.1) out of the previous transverse plane until it is parallel to the **left** costal arch. This positions it parallel to the course of the portal vein in the lesser omentum. Occasionally the transducer must be angled slightly cranially (Fig. 32.1b) to follow the course of the portal vein (11) from the porta hepatis all the way to the confluence (12 in Fig. 32.2b). The porta hepatis is best visualized in most patients on deep inspiration (don't forget the breathing command!), which displaces the liver and porta hepatis caudally and out from under the acoustic shadow of the ribs and lung.

Three hypoechoic vascular structures can be identified in the porta hepatis. The portal vein (11) normally lies immediately anterior to the obliquely sectioned (oval) inferior vena cava (16). The common bile duct (66) and common or proper hepatic artery (18) lie immediately anterior to the portal vein, just above it on the image. The hepatic artery and its branches are visualized only in segments because of their undulating course. These sectioned segments appear as round or oval structures (Fig. 32.2b) and must not be mistaken for periportal lymph nodes.

The common bile duct in a normal patient is often so narrow that it may only appear as a thin hypoechoic line or may not be identifiable at all. Its normal diameter should be less than 6 mm. In post-cholecystectomy patients, it partially assumes the reservoir function of the resected gallbladder and can dilate up to 9 mm without signifying cholestasis. Borderline dilation of the common bile duct or cholestasis, such as in obstruction caused by a stone, can then no longer unmistakably be differentiated from the adjacent blood vessels. In this situation, the entire length of all three vascular structures must be systematically visualized to determine their origin and with it their identity. The hepatic artery is traced to the celiac trunk, the portal vein to its confluence and to the splenic vein, and the common bile duct to the head of the pancreas. When visualizing the common bile duct, one can also identify or exclude intraductal stones (see p. 44). Color Doppler duplex sonography, if available, can be used as an alternate or supplementary modality to differentiate these vascular structures.

The normal diameter of the portal vein (11) measured perpendicular to its longitudinal axis at its widest point at the porta hepatis is usually less than 13 mm. Dilation should only be suspected where the diameter exceeds 15 mm. Measurements in between fall into the "gray area" of physiologic variation. Isolated dilation of the portal vein is a relatively unreliable criterion for portal hypertension. Positive evidence of portocaval collateral circulation is a more accurate criterion. The porta hepatis must be systematically scanned to detect atypical periportal vascular convolutions (see p. 33).

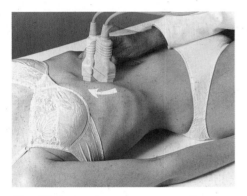

Fig. 32.1 a

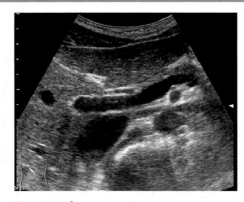

Fig. 32.1 b

Normal values of the porta hepatis:

Portal vein:	< 13 mm (maximum 15 mm)
Common bile duct:	< 6 mm (< 9 mm post-cholecystectomy)

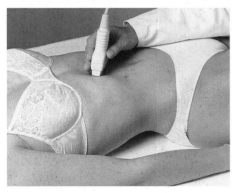

Fig. 32.2 a

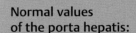

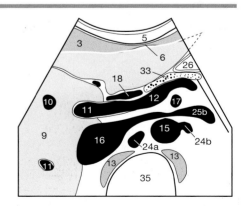

Fig. 32.2 b

Fig. 32.2 c

The most common cause of increasing pressure in the portal venous system is impaired drainage secondary to cirrhosis. Direct compression of the portal vein by an adjacent tumor is less common. Isolated compression of the splenic vein or superior mesenteric vein can occur in a pancreatic tumor without involvement of the portal vein. Dilation of the portal vein **(11)** to more than 15 mm in diameter suggests portal hypertension **(Fig. 33.1)**. The lumen of the portal vein is measured perpendicular to the vessel's longitudinal axis, which is usually oblique on the ultrasound image. The measurement should exclude the vascular wall.

Bear in mind that splenomegaly of other etiology can dilate the splenic vein to more than 12 mm or the portal vein to more than 15 mm even in the absence of portal hypertension.

Isolated dilation of the portal vein is an unreliable criterion for portal hypertension. Important additional criteria include congestive splenomegaly **(Fig. 72.2)**, ascites (see pp. 41, 60, 69), and above all portocaval anastomoses at the porta hepatis. These collaterals usually drain blood from the congested portal system via the greater curvature of the stomach and the dilated left gastric to the esophageal venous plexus. From there the blood drains via the azygos and hemiazygos veins into the superior vena cava. Possible clinical complications include bleeding esophageal varices.

Occasionally, small venous connections between the splenic hilum and left renal vein expand, allowing venous drainage directly into the inferior vena cava (spontaneous splenorenal shunt). A less common occurrence is recanalization of the umbilical vein, which courses along the margin of the ligamentum teres from the porta hepatis to the umbilicus (Cruveilhier–Baumgarten syndrome). Where this collateral circulation is well established **(Fig. 33.2)**, the often dilated umbilical vein can develop into a subcutaneous periumbilical venous plexus referred to as "caput medusae." When in doubt, color duplex sonography can be used to detect either a reduced flow rate or retrograde (hepatofugal) flow in the portal venous system.

Evaluation of the porta hepatis should not focus solely on the portal vein, but should specifically confirm or exclude enlarged periportal lymph nodes (**55** in **Fig. 33.3**). This requires systematic scanning of the periportal region. Inflammatory nodal enlargement frequently accompanies viral hepatitis, cholecystitis, or pancreatitis. Positive findings invariably require evaluation of other lymph node groups and measurement of spleen size to provide baseline data so that subsequent follow-up studies can provide valid information about progression or regression of the disorder.

Checklist for portal hypertension:

- Portocaval collaterals detected at the porta hepatis
- Diameter of portal vein at the porta hepatis ≥ 15 mm
- Dilation of splenic vein > 12 mm
- Splenomegaly
- Ascites detected
- Recanalized umbilical vein (Cruveilhier–Baumgarten syndrome)
- Esophageal varices (bleeding)

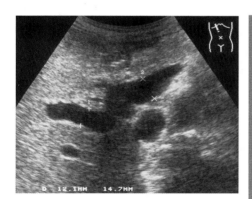

Fig. 33.1 a

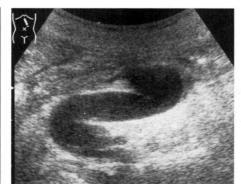

Fig. 33.2 a

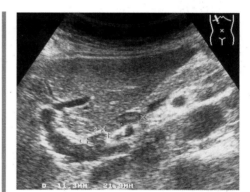

Fig. 33.3 a

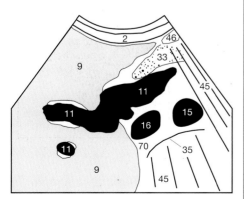

Fig. 33.1 b

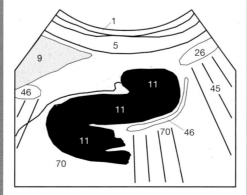

Fig. 33.2 b

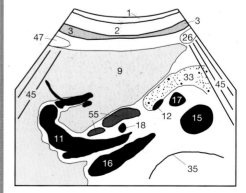

Fig. 33.3 b

After this lesson, we will have to add oblique planes to the more readily understandable sagittal and transverse planes we have been using. This makes identifying the individual structures in three-dimensional space considerably more demanding for the examiner. Do yourself a favor and do not begin Lesson 3 until you can easily answer all of the following questions, even if it requires some practice.

Here is a tip for time management: Do not spend more than two minutes on any one exercise (you will not retain anything after that anyway). Allow at least two hours between exercises and do other things in the interim (interval method). Correct your answers critically and do not give up too easily.

1. On a separate sheet of paper, please draw the approximate course of the most important upper abdominal blood vessels in relation to each other and to the pancreas. Do this entirely from memory without consulting this work-book or any other references. Label each structure with the customary abbreviations. Compare your drawing to **Figs. 27.2** and **27.3**. Consult the legends on the back cover flap to resolve anything you are uncertain about or have forgotten. Keep repeating this exercise with a little deter-mination until you can complete it without making any mistakes.

2. Consolidate your knowledge of tomographic anatomy by drawing (from memory, of course) the standard transverse planes through the celiac trunk and at the level where the renal veins cross. Compare your sketches with the drawings shown on page 114. You will only **permanently** remember those structures whose contours you can draw correctly in both position and size.

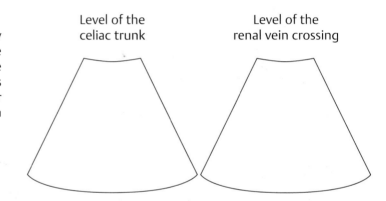

Level of the   Level of the
celiac trunk   renal vein crossing

3. How does the echogenicity of the pancreatic parenchyma change with advancing age and in obesity? What trick do you know to improve visualization of the tail of the pancreas? What other imaging modalities are available for evaluating the pancreas?

4. Name every vessel and every other structure on the image shown in **Fig. 34.1**. Which vessel appears dilated or congested? What could cause this? Is this a pathologic finding? The solution can be found on page 123.

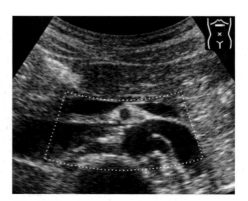

Fig. 34.1

Lesson 3 covers the liver and gallbladder. Both organs should be scanned systematically in two planes with the **entire** examination performed in deep inspiration. We recommend always following a standard system: Begin in the sagittal plane using the inferior vena cava as a demarcation line as shown in **Fig. 21.3**. From there, scan laterally to the left and back to visualize the left hepatic lobe. After pausing to let the patient exhale and take another breath, continue by scanning the right hepatic lobe the same way, slowly and continuously sweeping the transducer **(Fig. 35.1a)**. The main problem for the examiner is visualizing the cranial subdiaphragmatic segments of the liver. The patient must inhale as deeply as possible and the transducer must be tilted to the proper angle **(Fig. 35.1b)**. Because of the larger size of the right lobe, this maneuver must usually be performed once for the cranial segments and then, after allowing the patient to catch his or her breath, repeated for the caudal segments. Remember to

reduce the magnification to allow you to evaluate the posterior segments of the liver as well. Keep in mind that the portal venous branches **(11)** in the hepatic parenchyma **(9)** are always surrounded by a hyperechoic rim ("embankment") because of the adjacent biliary ducts, arteries, and periportal connective tissue. Depending on the insonation angle, the hepatic veins **(10)** are usually visualized without a hyperechoic border (which can be seen only with a 90° insonation angle).

Measuring the size of the liver has fallen from favor in recent years because of the poor reliability of such measurements. Typically the craniocaudal and anteroposterior diameter were measured in the sagittal plane along the right midclavicular line **(Fig. 35.2)**. The normal craniocaudal diameter measures between 11 and 15 cm in adults but varies greatly with the depth of inspiration because of the elastic adaption of the hepatic parenchyma **(9)** to the shape of the chest cavity. It is more helpful to evaluate the inferior angle of the right lobe, which should be less than 45°. This angle appears rounded in a congested liver or in hepatomegaly of any other etiology. The lateral inferior angle of the left lobe should be less than 30° and is normally more acute than the caudal margin of the liver.

The gallbladder **(14)** on the caudal margin of the liver can be evaluated at the same time. The gallbladder should be evaluated in a fasting patient **(Fig. 35.3)** as it is then easier to assess the wall thickness **(80)**, which should not exceed 4 mm. Postprandial contraction of the gallbladder does not allow one to reliably exclude edematous thickening of the wall, stones, polyps, or tumors (see pp. 45, 46).

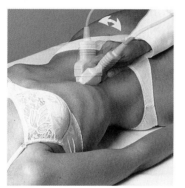

Fig. 35.1 a

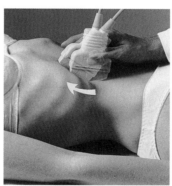

Fig. 35.1 b

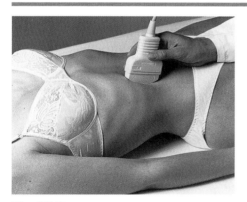

Fig. 35.2 a

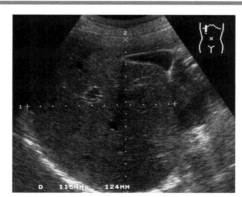

Fig. 35.2 b

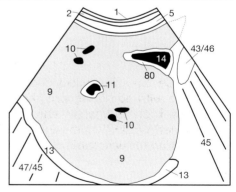

Fig. 35.2 c

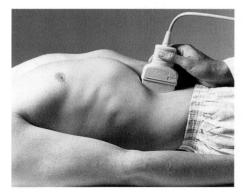

Fig. 35.3 a

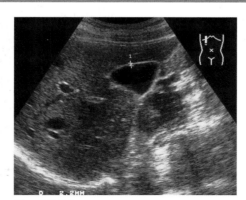

Fig. 35.3 b

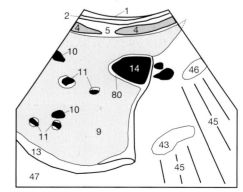

Fig. 35.3 c

After the liver has been scanned in the sagittal plane, the left lobe is now systematically scanned craniocaudally in the transverse plane to detect any possible focal masses. For practical reasons it is best to visualize the right lobe in a subcostal oblique plane parallel to the right costal arch (**Fig. 36.1**). What mistake is commonly made when holding the probe? The answer is in the lower left-hand corner of this page.

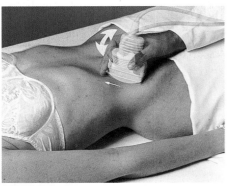

Fig. 36.1

Hepatic Venous Star

This right subcostal oblique plane (**Fig. 36.2a**) is especially useful for visualizing long segments of the hepatic veins (**10**) as far as their confluence with the oval cross section of the obliquely visualized inferior vena cava. This long straight course of the hepatic veins is typical and changes only in the presence of focal intrahepatic masses or right heart failure.

Right Heart Failure

Where the inferior vena cava exhibits a borderline diameter and the vena cava collapse test during forced inspiration is inconclusive, the diameter of the peripheral hepatic veins can provide additional evidence to confirm or exclude right heart failure. The maximum diameter of a peripheral hepatic vein (in the left upper corner of the image) should not exceed 6 mm. Measuring the central hepatic veins closer to the vena cava (**16**) is problematic due to the wide range of physiologic variation; 10 to 12 mm can be perfectly normal at this location. **Fig. 36.3** shows the typical picture of overt right heart failure with congested, engorged hepatic veins and an engorged inferior vena cava (**16**).

Please note that in this plane the right hepatic vein lies perpendicular to the direction of the sound waves and can therefore exhibit a thin hyperechoic wall otherwise seen only in the portal venous branches (**11** in **Fig. 36.2b**). This plane is also very well suited for evaluating the hepatic veins with color duplex studies where venous thrombosis is suspected. In any case, be alert to diminished vascularity in the peripheral segments of the liver as an indirect sign of cirrhotic transformation of the hepatic parenchyma.

A right pleural effusion can also be confirmed in this imaging plane behind (on the image beneath) the hyperechoic diaphragm (**13**). At this site there are normally only acoustic shadows (**45**) behind pulmonary air (**47**) or a mirror image artifact caused by the hepatic parenchyma (**9**).

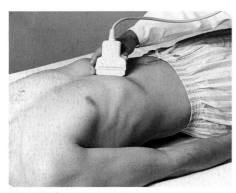

Fig. 36.2 a

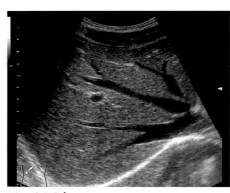

Fig. 36.2 b

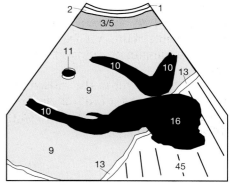

Fig. 36.2 c

Normal Values:
Hepatic veins: < 6 mm
(periphery)

Answer to Fig. 36.1:
The transducer is positioned too far laterally and caudally. It should be moved medially and closer to the costal arch (see small arrow).

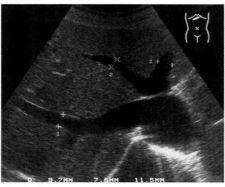

Fig. 36.3 a

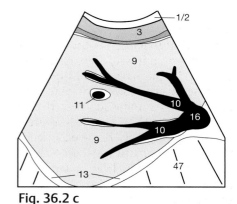

Fig. 36.3 b

Systematic examination of the liver can reveal normal variants that mimic focal masses. For instance, athletic patients may occasionally exhibit hyperechoic (↓) structures along the dome of the liver that appear to extend from the diaphragm **(13)** and indent the hepatic parenchyma **(Fig. 37.1)**. These apparent lesions represent thickened muscular bands in the diaphragm that extend from the bare area of the liver to the caudal ribs and lumbar vertebrae, creating a series of cordlike impressions in the liver.

They have no clinical significance and must not be mistaken for pathologic processes. Such a muscular band **(13)** may occur in isolation **(Fig. 37.2)** and be projected as a mirror image artifact **(51)** on the pulmonary side **(47)** of the diaphragm (see p. 17).

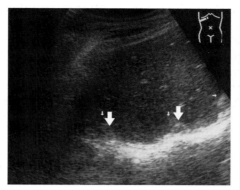

Fig. 37.1 a

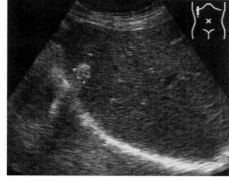

Fig. 37.2 a

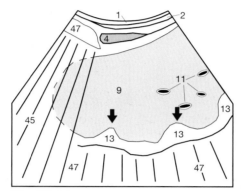

Fig. 37.1 b

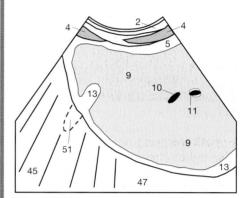

Fig. 37.2 b

Fatty Liver

A fatty liver (hepatic steatosis) is characterized by diffusely increased echogenicity in the liver **(Fig. 37.3)**. This increase in echogenicity is best demonstrated by comparison with the adjacent kidney **(29)**. Normally there is hardly any difference in the echogenicity of the two organs (see **Fig. 47.3**). In severe cases of fatty liver, sound reflection from the hepatic tissue **(9)** can be so pronounced as to effectively prevent evaluation of the deeper layers of the liver. **Fig. 37.4** shows acoustic enhancement **(70)** immediately posterior to the gallbladder **(14)**. However, the posterior segments of the liver are no longer visualized despite depth gain compensation.

Do you remember the reason for the phenomenon of distal acoustic enhancement? If not, go back to page 16 and reread that section.

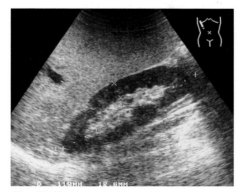

Fig. 37.3 a

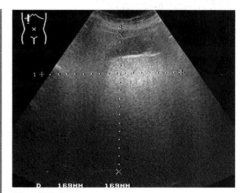

Fig. 37.4 a

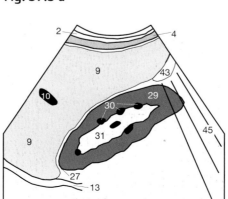

Fig. 37.3 b

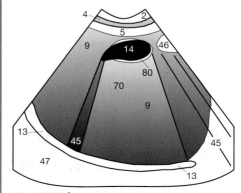

Fig. 37.4 b

Focal Fatty Infiltration

Fatty liver is not necessarily a diffuse process involving the entire organ; infiltration can also be confined to individual segments of the liver. Such focal fatty infiltration (63) shows a predilection for the gallbladder bed and the area anterior to the portal vein (11). These zones of increased fat deposition are more hyperechoic than the rest of the parenchyma (9) and are invariably sharply demarcated. They can exhibit bizarre geographic configurations (Fig. 38.1) but lack any signs of a mass effect. Adjacent hepatic veins (10) and portal vein branches (11) are **not** displaced.

These areas of focal fatty infiltration must be distinguished from the falciform ligament (8) whose connective tissue and surrounding fat can appear as a similar sharply demarcated structure interrupting the normal hepatic parenchyma (Fig. 38.2).

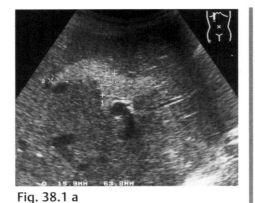

Fig. 38.1 a

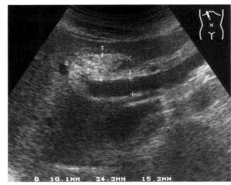

Fig. 38.2 a

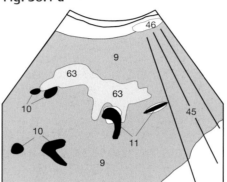

Fig. 38.1 b

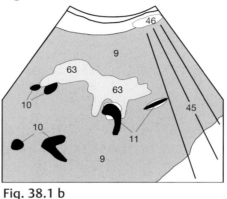

Fig. 38.2 b

Focal Sparing in Fatty Infiltration

Fatty infiltration can also spare individual segments of the liver, creating focal areas of reduced infiltration (62). These zones often occur in the immediate vicinity of the portal vein and gallbladder (14 in Fig. 38.4). The important thing is that here, too, there are no signs of a mass effect. Adjacent hepatic veins (10) are not displaced (Fig. 38.3) but exhibit their normal straight course. Peripheral areas of focal sparing do not cause any outward bulging or project into the gallbladder as is often observed with focal malignancies.

The branches of the portal vein (11) can be distinguished from hepatic veins by a hyperechoic border. This "embankment" is caused by impedance mismatches between the walls of the portal venous branches, the accompanying biliary ducts, and the arteries. The "embankment" (5) often appears thicker in the vicinity of the porta hepatis (Fig. 38.2) and should not be mistaken for focal fatty infiltration. Because the hepatic veins course through the parenchyma (9) without accompanying arteries, they do not exhibit this impedance mismatch. The vascular wall produces a bright echo only when major hepatic veins are visualized perpendicular to the sound beam (see p. 36).

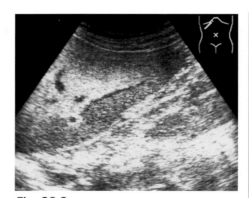

Fig. 38.3 a

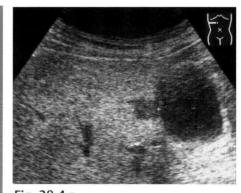

Fig. 38.4 a

Fig. 38.3 b

Fig. 38.4 b

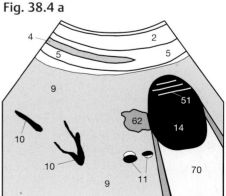

The most common focal lesions in the liver are benign cysts **(64)**. These can be congenital (dysontogenetic) or acquired. The latter can be distinguished from congenital dilation of the bile ducts (Caroli syndrome) because they contain no bile but only serous fluid **(Fig. 39.1)**. Because they are filled with homogeneous fluid, they are anechoic unless bleeding into a cyst has occurred. Congenital liver cysts are usually of no clinical significance.

Cyst Criteria

The following features make it easier to differentiate benign cysts from other hypoechoic masses: anechoic content, spherical shape, sharp and smooth demarcation, and distal acoustic enhancement in the case of larger cysts (see p. 16). Occasionally there are edge shadows (p. 17) and accentuated entry and exit echoes (where the incident sound waves hit the cysts at a 90° angle). The internal echoes occurring in hemorrhagic cysts can present diagnostic difficulties. These cysts can also exhibit indentations or fine septa. Where this is the case, differential diagnosis must exclude parasitic infestation of the liver **(Fig. 39.4)**.

The most common cause of parasitic liver disease is enteral infection with the dog tapeworm (Echinococcus cysticus), which characteristically produces several daughter cysts within a larger cyst. Such cysts should not be aspirated to avoid rupture and subsequent seeding of the abdominal cavity with the pathogen. The less common fox tapeworm (Echinococcus alveolaris) is difficult to identify on ultrasound scans. Typical findings include a mixed solid, liquid, and cystic mass **(54 in Fig. 39.4a)**. It is virtually impossible to distinguish these lesions from a primary carcinoma of the liver, a metastasis **(Fig. 42.3)**, or an abscess.

Hepatic hemangiomas (61) on the other hand are homogeneously hyperechoic (bright) in comparison with the adjacent hepatic parenchyma **(9)**, are sharply demarcated, and lack a hypoechoic rim **(Fig. 39.2)**. They typically occur in the vicinity of a draining hepatic vein **(10)** as in **Fig. 39.3**. Hepatic hemangiomas are usually small **(Fig. 39.2)** but can also be multifocal and quite large. Larger hemangiomas often become inhomogeneous, making them difficult to distinguish from other tumors. A supplementary CT scan is then indicated (see next page).

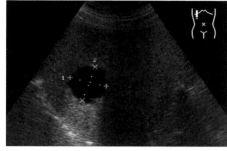

Fig. 39.1 a

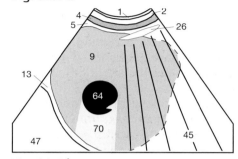

Fig. 39.1 b

Checklist of Cyst Criteria
- Spherical shape
- Anechoic contents
- Sharply demarcated
- Distal acoustic enhancement
- Edge shadow
- Accentuated entry and exit echoes

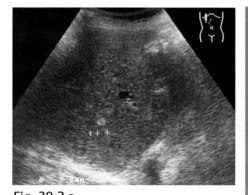

Fig. 39.2 a

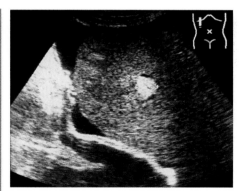

Fig. 39.3 a

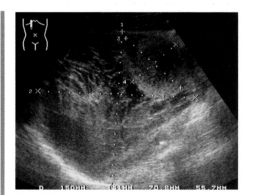

Fig. 39.4 a

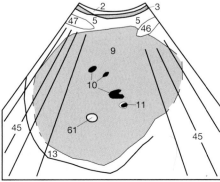

Fig. 39.2 b

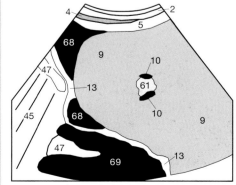

Fig. 39.3 b

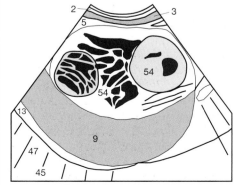

Fig. 39.4 b

Inflammatory processes in the liver can be caused by cholangitis, fungal disease in immunosuppressed patients, or hematogenous spread of pathogens. Morphologic findings on ultrasound are highly variable.

Depending on the stage of the lesion and the patient's immune status, liver abscesses can exhibit central liquefaction **(Fig. 40.2)**, inhomogeneous areas with a hypoechoic rim, or even hyperechoic structures **(Fig. 40.1)**. The variable appearance of abscesses makes them difficult to differentiate from focal nodular hyperplasia (FNH, **Fig. 40.3**), which can also appear inhomogeneous, like malignant tumors of the liver. FNH is a primary benign liver tumor that occurs more frequently in women taking oral contraceptives. Special contrast studies often show a typical stellate pattern in the center during the early arterial phase **(Fig. 40.4)**.

When in doubt, a spiral CT study can distinguish these lesions from large, inhomogeneous hemangiomas. Hemangiomas show an "iris sign" after a bolus injection of contrast agent as the enhancement progresses from the outside to the inside like a closing iris, producing a target sign **(Fig. 40.5)**.

Liver tumors can produce an intrahepatic mass that compresses adjacent hepatic tissue. Cholestasis resulting from compression of adja-

cent bile ducts can be temporarily relieved via a stent into the duodenum or via a percutaneous drainage catheter into a collection bag. The effectiveness of an indwelling drainage catheter **(59)** can be readily evaluated by noninvasive ultrasound follow-up studies **(Fig. 40.1)**.

Air in the Bile Ducts

Occasionally fine gas bubbles **(60)** can be observed in the bile ducts **(66)** secondary to infections or after ERCP, papillotomy, or creation of a biliary-enteric anastomosis **(Fig. 40.2)** even without infection. The acronym **ERCP** stands for endoscopic retrograde cholangiopancreatography. Via the operating channel of an endoscope advanced through the duodenum to the major papilla, a second "baby" endoscope is advanced in retrograde fashion into the orifice of the distal common bile duct. A papillotomy is an incision into a scarred stenosed papilla.

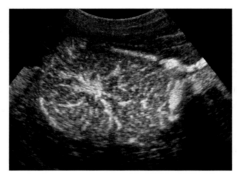

Fig. 40.4 (Prof. Dietrich, Univ. of Frankfurt)

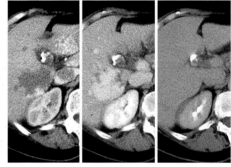

Fig. 40.5

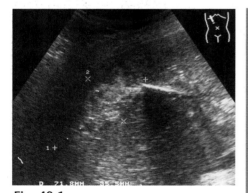

Fig. 40.1 a

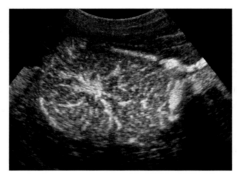

Fig. 40.2 a

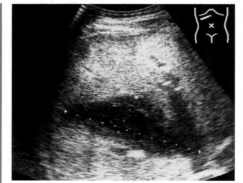

Fig. 40.3 a

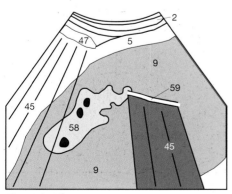

Fig. 40.1 b

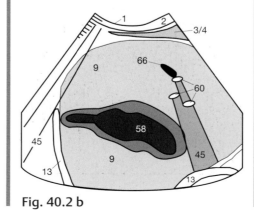

Fig. 40.2 b

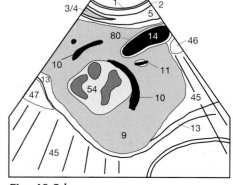

Fig. 40.3 b

In addition to chronic alcohol abuse, cirrhosis may occur as a late sequela of viral inflammation of the liver (hepatitis), metabolic disorders, or exposure to environmental toxins. Latent cirrhosis without signs of hepatic decompensation can be present in the absence of morphologic changes on ultrasound studies. Consequently, cirrhosis cannot be excluded by ultrasound alone. However, there are several criteria for more advanced stages of cirrhosis.

Cirrhosis Criteria

Whereas a normal liver (9) exhibits a thin hyperechoic capsule along its border (see **Fig. 35.3**), the surface of the cirrhotic liver is often irregular with small undulations or bumps. This causes increased scattering so that echoes reflected from the capsule are lost to the transducer. The capsule is visualized only partially or not at all. The absence of a capsular line is best appreciated where ascites (68) is simultaneously present (**Fig. 41.1**). Another characteristic finding in cirrhosis is diminished peripheral vascularity (**Fig. 41.1**). The hepatic veins that are still visualized often exhibit variable caliber and wider confluence angles (>45°). Normal hepatic veins (10) course largely in a straight line, join each other at an acute angle, and can be traced into the periphery of the liver as in **Fig. 36.2**.

The portal venous branches close to the porta hepatis often show a pronounced "embankment" and abrupt changes in caliber occasionally referred to as a "pruned portal tree." Regenerating nodules are often isoechoic to normal parenchyma and can only be inferred from the displacement of adjacent vessels. A thickened biconvex liver, decreased pliability when pressed with the transducer, and thickening and enlargement of the left hepatic or caudate lobe all suggest cirrhosis.

Complications of Cirrhosis

Possible sequelae of cirrhosis include portal hypertension (see p. 33), ascites (68), and malignant liver tumors (54) that develop in the setting of chronic cirrhosis (**Fig. 41.2**). Therefore it is important to inspect every cirrhotic liver carefully and thoroughly for focal masses. Shrinkage of the liver (**Fig. 41.2**) occurs only in the late stage of cirrhosis. Occasionally the tumors are isoechoic to the rest of the hepatic parenchyma (9) and can only be inferred from the displacement of adjacent hepatic veins (10 in **Fig. 41.3**).

Checklist of Cirrhosis Criteria

- Absence of thin hyperechoic capsule line
- Diminished peripheral vascularity
- Widened angle of the hepatic veins > 45°
- Abrupt caliber changes of the portal vein
- Possible enhanced "embankment" in the portal vein
- Regenerating nodules with displaced vessels

Additional Findings in the Late Stage

- Rounded organ shape (obtuse marginal angles)
- Shrinkage of the liver
- Signs of portal hypertension

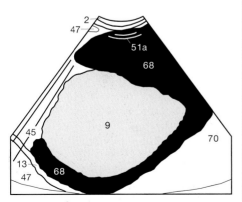

Fig. 41.1 a

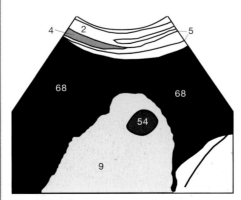

Fig. 41.2 a

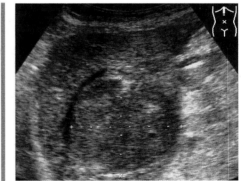

Fig. 41.3 a

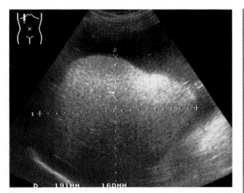

Fig. 41.1 b

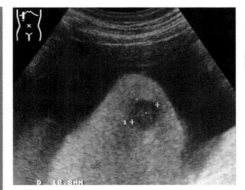

Fig. 41.2 b

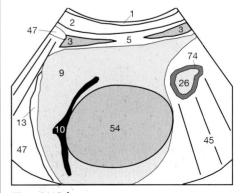

Fig. 41.3 b

Malignant secondary tumors (metastases) arise in the liver not only from hematogenous seeding of gastrointestinal tumors via the portal vein, but are often observed with breast and bronchial carcinomas. Ultrasound findings are, unfortunately, highly variable. Colorectal carcinomas usually produce hyperechoic metastases **(56)** in the liver **(Fig. 42.2)** because the relatively slow growth of the metastasis means that pathologic vessels can develop within it. Rapidly growing metastases of bronchial or breast carcinomas consist almost entirely of tumor cells and therefore tend to be hypoechoic.

Because of the many mixed types of metastases it is not possible to reliably correlate metastases with a certain type of primary tumor, despite the fact that the visualization of vascular architecture and evaluation of the elasticity of focal lesions now possible on color duplex studies will add a promising new dimension to differential diagnostic evaluation.

Metastases **(56)** typically exhibit a hypoechoic (dark) rim or halo as seen in **Figs. 42.1** and **42.2**. This halo can represent either a perifocal edema or a zone of active proliferation. Metastases can also exhibit central necrosis in the form of cystic liquefaction due to rapid growth or chemotherapy **(Fig. 42.3)**.

Larger metastases often show the characteristics of a mass, displacing adjacent vessels and occasionally causing compression of bile ducts leading to regional intrahepatic cholestasis **(Fig. 43.2)**. Metastases located near the surface of the liver can show focal expansion of the liver contour that is readily visible on laparoscopy.

Chemotherapy can induce variable signs of tumor regression depending on the therapeutic effect. These include inhomogeneous scars, calcifications, or partial cystic transformation of the metastasis. Such regressive metastases or small nodular metastases can be difficult to distinguish from cirrhotic processes. Follow-up studies to evaluate growth are crucial as are ultrasound or CT-guided needle biopsies. Multiple metastases of differing size and echogenicity suggest hematogenous spread at different times.

Quiz – Test Yourself:
Use the images on this page to test your basic knowledge. Do you remember why hypoechoic (dark) bands **(45)** traverse the liver in **Fig. 42.1** and why the region between them **(70)** appears slightly more hyperechoic (brighter) than the rest of the hepatic parenchyma **(9)**? Remember: The gallbladder **(14)** lies between the two artifacts and the transducer and the sound beam strikes its wall **(80)** tangentially. If you still cannot think of a satisfactory explanation, please go back and study pages 16 and 17.
On the subject of images: Did you not notice three pages back in **Fig. 39.3a** the anechoic (black) areas of the image, which physiologically cannot appear that way? If you have not already found a solution, please have another look at the image. You will find the solution to this puzzle on page 125.

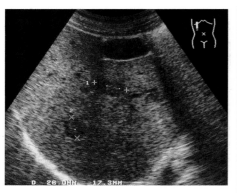

Fig. 42.1 a

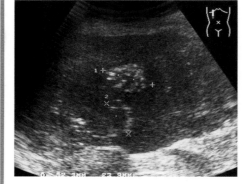

Fig. 42.2 a

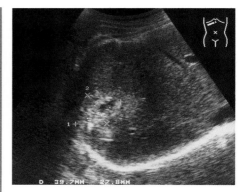

Fig. 42.3 a

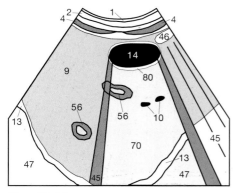

Fig. 42.1 b

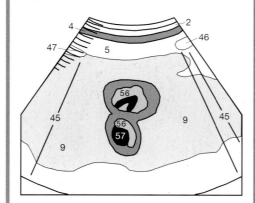

Fig. 42.2 b

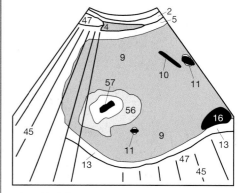

Fig. 42.3 b

At the level of the lesser omentum at the porta hepatis, the common bile duct **(66)** normally measures up to 6 mm in diameter, although diameters between 7 and 9 mm are still within the normal range, particularly in post-cholecystectomy patients **(Fig.43.1)**. The bile duct is almost invariably visualized anterolateral to (above) the portal vein **(11)** (see p. 32). Even when the distal common bile duct near the head of the pancreas is obscured by duodenal air (see **Fig. 29.1**), ultrasound can reliably differentiate proximal obstructive jaundice (such as from hepatic metastases with intrahepatic biliary obstruction) from distal obstructive jaundice (such as from a gallstone lodged at the papilla or a carcinoma of the head of the pancreas). In a proximal obstruction, neither the gallbladder **(14)** nor the common bile duct are distended.

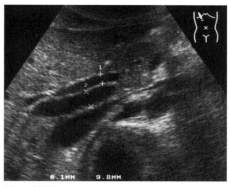
Fig. 43.1 a

Obstructive Cholestasis
The small intrahepatic bile ducts course parallel to the branches of the portal vein **(11)** and are normally visualized as fine structures or not at all. In obstructive cholestasis these dilated ducts are visible alongside the portal veins, creating a "double barrel shotgun sign" **(Figs. 43.2 and 44.3)**. In about 90% of all cases, ultrasound can distinguish obstructive cholestasis (with dilation of the bile ducts) from hepatocellular cholestasis (without obstruction).

Mechanical obstruction **(Fig. 43.2)** typically leads to dilation of the intrahepatic bile ducts **(66)** in a pattern resembling the antlers of a deer. This may be accompanied by crystalline precipitation **(67)** of cholesterol, calcium, and/or bilirubin depending on the specific composition of the bile. This "sludge" **(67)** can also occur secondary to prolonged parenteral nutrition without biliary obstruction.

Before diagnosing the presence of "sludge," you should exclude a section thickness artifact (see p. 16) by verifying findings in several imaging planes and repositioning the patient. When in doubt, attempt to shake up the sludge with the transducer under direct visualization. In obstructive cholestasis, **ERCP** (**e**ndoscopic **r**etrograde **c**holangio**p**ancreatography) can be performed to place a catheter **(59)** to drain the bile into the duodenum **(Fig. 43.4)**. Alternatively, a percutaneous transhepatic catheter can be placed to drain the bile into an external collection bag.

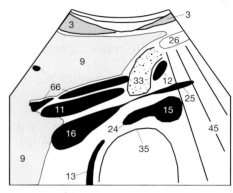
Fig. 43.1 b

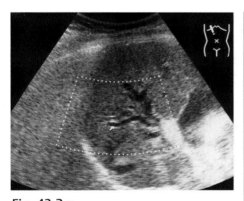
Fig. 43.2 a

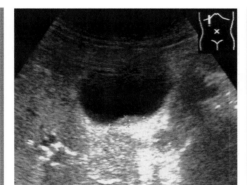
Fig. 43.3 a

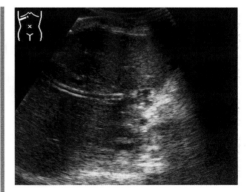
Fig. 43.4 a

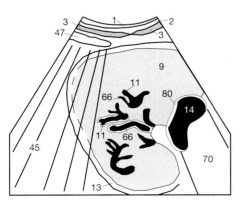
Fig. 43.2 b

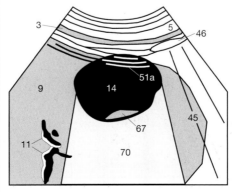
Fig. 43.3 b

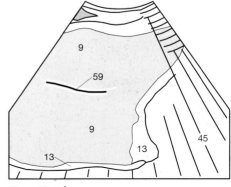
Fig. 43.4 b

Stones in the gallbladder (gallstones) form because of altered composition of the excreted bile. Depending on their composition, gallstones **(49)** can be nearly completely permeable for sound waves and therefore visible on ultrasound **(Fig. 44.3)**, they can float within the gallbladder (cholesterol stones), or their calcium content can make them so reflective that the stone cannot be visualized in its entirety **(Fig. 44.1)**.

A stone is easily differentiated from a polyp **(65)** when it can be dislodged from the gallbladder wall **(80)** by repositioning the patient **(Fig. 44.2)** or mobilizing it with the transducer. However, some stones adhere to the gallbladder wall due to previous inflammatory processes or become lodged in the infundibulum, rendering differential diagnosis difficult.
Acoustic shadowing **(45)** behind such a lesion **(Figs. 44.1** and **44.3)** also suggests a stone. Here, it is important to distinguish an edge shadow of the gallbladder wall **(45 in Fig. 44.2)** from the acoustic shadow of a stone (see p. 17) to avoid any misinterpretation. **Fig. 44.2** shows mural polyps without acoustic shadowing but with adjacent edge shadows. Such polyps should be monitored to exclude progressive growth. This allows early detection of a malignant process. One may also opt for prophylactic surgical removal to preclude malignant transformation.

Intrahepatic cholestasis **(Fig. 43.2)** is not necessarily the result of bile duct compression by a malignant tumor. Gallstones **(49)** in the intrahepatic ducts **(66 in Fig. 44.3)** can also be the cause of the obstruction.

The prevalence of gallstones is about 15% in the German population, with older women more often affected. As about 80% of patients with gallstones remain asymptomatic, detection of gallstones is only clinically significant in the presence of complications (cholecystitis, cholangitis, colic, or cholestasis due to impacted stones). Common risk factors are listed in **Table 44.4**. Depending on the specific case, removal of the stone can be attempted by e**x**tracorporeal **s**hock **w**ave **l**ithotripsy (**ESWL**), ERCP (see p. 40), or surgery. The composition of the bile can also be influenced by medication and change of diet, which causes some stones to regress.

Note the thin, single-layer, hyperechoic line of the wall **(80)** of the two gallbladders **(14)** shown in **Figs. 44.1** and **44.2**. There is no detectable inflammatory thickening of the gallbladder wall. Ultrasound examination of the gallbladder should always be performed in the fasting patient to facilitate detection of wall thickening or intraluminal processes. Postprandial contraction of the gallbladder precludes an adequate evaluation of its lumen. Typical images of inflammation of the gallbladder (cholecystitis) are shown on the next page.

Risk factors for gall stones: 5 x "F"
• female
• forty
• fertile (mother)
• fat (obesity)
• fair (blonde)

Table 44.4

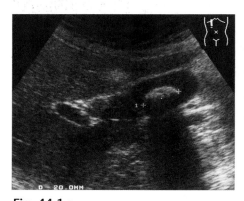

Fig. 44.1 a

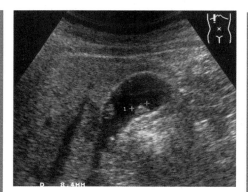

Fig. 44.2 a

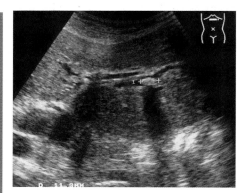

Fig. 44.3 a

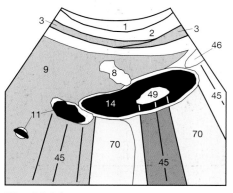

Fig. 44.1 b

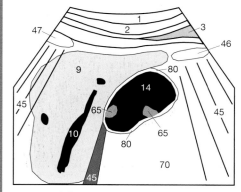

Fig. 44.2 b

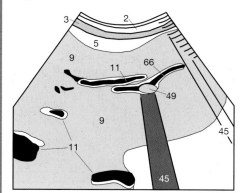

Fig. 44.3 b

The normal preprandial gallbladder **(14)** has a thin, single-layer wall **(80)** less than 4 mm thick **(Fig. 45.3)**. Cholecystitis is most often caused by stones **(49)** in the gallbladder **(14)**. A tender gallbladder can be the only finding in early cholecystitis, but this is soon followed by inflammatory edema with thickening of the gallbladder wall **(80)**, whose multilayered structure then becomes clearly visible **(Fig. 45.1)**.

Thickening of the gallbladder wall is also seen in ascites **(68)** but without inflammatory infiltration. This can also be caused by right heart failure or hypoalbuminemia **(Fig. 45.2)**.

An additional finding indicative of acute inflammation **(Table 45.4)** is a rim of fluid around the gallbladder **(68)**. In some cases, fluid is also detected in the hepatorenal fossa (pouch of Morrison) between the caudal margin of the liver and the right kidney (see **Fig. 112.5**). Finally, the outline of the gallbladder can become blurred along the adjacent hepatic parenchyma **(9)**. A transverse diameter of the gallbladder of more than 4 cm indicates hydrops. A more reliable sign is the change from a typical pear shape to a biconvex spherical shape.

Prompt detection of gas within the gallbladder or in its wall (mural emphysema) is more important as infection with a gas-forming organism has a poor prognosis and is associated with a higher risk of acute perforation. Chronic cholecystitis can lead to a contracted gallbladder or porcelain gallbladder. The two forms are often difficult to differentiate on ultrasound. Because a completely calcified gallbladder wall can reflect sound waves like air in the hepatic flexure of the colon, it is easy to miss a porcelain gallbladder on ultrasound. The diagnosis is often made on the basis of clinical findings or a supplemental CT study in these cases.

The postprandial gallbladder in its contracted, empty state often exhibits a kink reminiscent of a beret **(Fig. 45.3)**. The concave side can show an indentation (⤵) that should not be misinterpreted as a septum.

Checklist for Acute Cholecystitis
• Thickened, multilayered wall
• Fluid rim around gallbladder
• Indistinct border between gallbladder and liver
• Wall thickness ≥ 4 mm (preprandial)   ≥ 7 mm (postprandial)
• Tenderness to palpation with probe   in right midclavicular line
• Hyperperfusion on color duplex sonography

Table 45.4

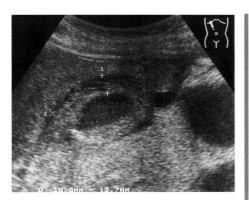

Fig. 45.1 a

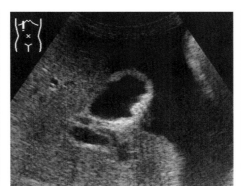

Fig. 45.2 a

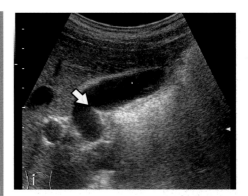

Fig. 45.3 a

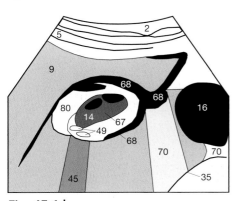

Fig. 45.1 b

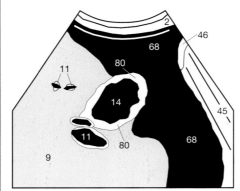

Fig. 45.2 b

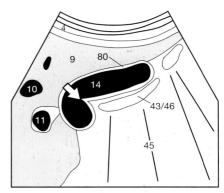

Fig. 45.3 b

Liver and Gallbladder: Quiz for Self Evaluation

Please take this quiz to test your command of the material presented in Lesson 3. You will find the answers to the questions on the preceding pages and the answers to the image quiz on page 123. Check the answers only after you have worked through all questions. Getting the answers too early ruins the suspense and defeats the purpose of the quiz.

1. Repeat the drawing exercise for the standard imaging plane of the porta hepatis. Where are hepatic artery and bile duct in relation to the portal vein and inferior vena cava? Compare your drawing with **Fig. 32.2c**.

2. What is the name of the imaging plane that visualizes the hepatic venous star? How do you hold the transducer to obtain this plane? Draw the corresponding body markers and draw the appearance of the hepatic venous star. What measurements can you make at which locations? For what purpose?

3. Write down six characteristics of portal hypertension and eight criteria of cirrhosis of the liver. Compare your answers with the checklists on pages 33 and 41, and repeat this exercise over the next few days until you remember every finding (leave time to rest in between!).

4. Do you remember the sites of predilection for focal fatty infiltration and focal areas of reduced fatty infiltration of the liver? How can you distinguish these processes from hepatic malignancies?

5. Review the following three ultrasound images. Write down the imaging planes, the organs and vessels visualized, and your differential diagnosis. Include **all** changes and your interpretation as some images include **several** pathologic processes.

6. What is the maximum diameter of the common bile duct? Above what diameter in mm would you suspect obstructive cholestasis?

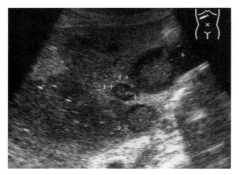

Fig. 46.1

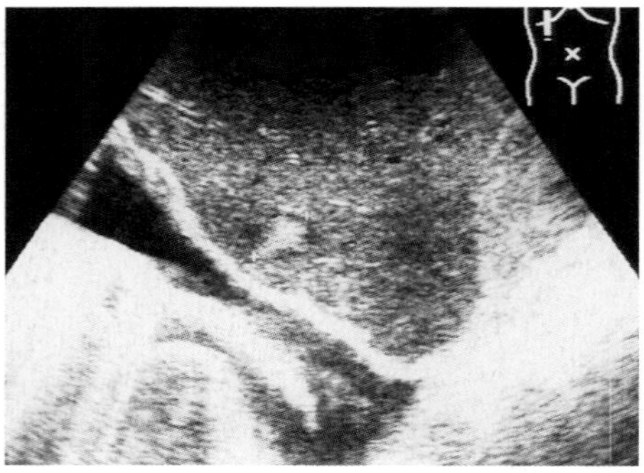

Fig. 46.2

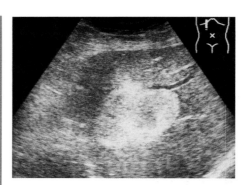

Fig. 46.3

7. Write down several differential diagnoses for **Fig. 46.4**. The solution is on page 123.

Fig. 46.4

Q

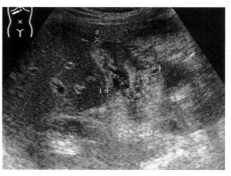

The right kidney can be well visualized in the longitudinal plane through the liver along the axillary line with the patient positioned supine and taking a deep breath (Fig. 47.2a). Alternatively, the transducer can be placed parallel to the intercostal spaces with the patient in the left lateral decubitus position (Fig. 47.1a). Scan each kidney thoroughly in two planes. The left kidney can be visualized in the longitudinal and transverse planes with the patient supine or in the right lateral decubitus position. Deep inspiration should displace the kidney caudally 3–7 cm to the level of the psoas major muscle (44). This displacement places the kidneys in a better acoustic window between the ribs and intestinal air.

Normally, the parenchyma of the right kidney is isoechoic to hepatic parenchyma (Fig. 47.3). It should be at least 1.3 cm thick. The hypoechoic medullary pyramids (30) are visualized in the typical longitudinal plane (Fig. 47.2) as a "string

of pearls" along the border between the outer parenchyma (29) and the hyperechoic central renal caliceal system. They should not be mistaken for anechoic cysts or renal calices. The central region of the kidney appears hyperechoic because of the many impedance mismatches between the walls of vascular structures, connective tissue, and fat.

The right renal hilum with the renal vein (25) extending to the inferior vena cava (16) is well visualized in the transverse plane (Fig. 47.3). Be alert to hypoechoic masses within the hyperechoic suprarenal fat capsule at the upper pole of the kidney (27) as these suggest adrenal tumors. An important measure of chronic kidney damage is the ratio of the thickness of the hypoechoic peripheral parenchyma to the hyperechoic renal pelvis in the center. This parenchyma to pelvis (PP) index increases with age (see table):

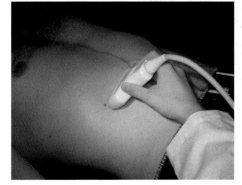

Fig. 47.1 a

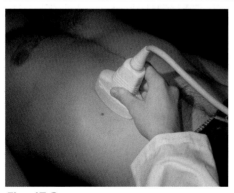

Fig. 47.1 b

Checklist of Normal Renal Values	
Kidney length:	10 – 12 cm
Kidney width:	4 – 6 cm
Respiratory mobility:	3 – 7 cm
Width of parenchyma:	1.3 – 2.5 cm
PP index, age < 30 years	> 1.6 : 1
PP index, age 30–60 years	1.2–1.6 : 1
PP index, age > 60 years	1.1 : 1

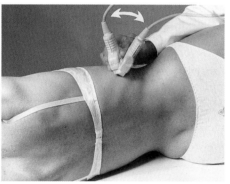

Fig. 47.2 a

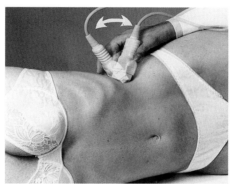

Fig. 47.2 b

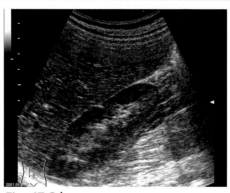

Fig. 47.2 c

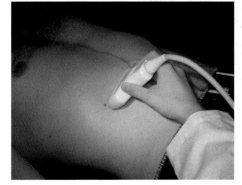

Fig. 47.3 a

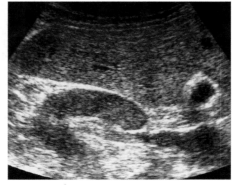

Fig. 47.3 b

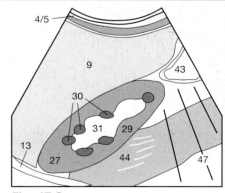

Fig. 47.3 c

Normal Variants

The normal shape of the kidney **(Fig. 47.2)** can exhibit several developmental variants. Hyperplastic columns of Bertin can protrude from the parenchyma **(29)** into the renal pelvis **(31)**. These columns are isoechoic to the rest of the parenchyma. An isoechoic parenchymal bridge can completely divide the renal pelvis, or partial or complete renal duplication **(Fig. 48.1)** may be present with separate ureters and blood supply for each moiety.

At first glance, a horseshoe kidney with prevertebral bridges can be misinterpreted as a preaortic lymphoma or thrombosed aortic aneurysm. An undulating kidney surface due to persisting fetal lobulation is occasionally observed in children and young adults. Although slightly domed, the surface itself is smooth. There may be fine indentations between the medullary pyramids. These indentations must be differentiated from the more triangular scars occurring secondary to renal infarcts (see **Fig. 56.3**), which are most often found in older patients with renal artery stenosis or suprarenal aortic aneurysm.

About 10% of all patients show localized parenchymal thickening along the lateral border of the left kidney, usually caudal to the adjacent lower pole of the spleen. The "dromedary hump" is a normal bulge that can be difficult to differentiate from a tumor.

Renal Cysts

Dysontogenetic cysts **(64)** are usually anechoic as in the liver (see p. 39). Above a certain size they show distal acoustic enhancement **(70)** as in **Fig. 48.2**. Do you remember the other criteria for differentiating cysts from hypoechoic renal tumors in obese patients? If not, you know where to find them.

Peripheral cysts lying on the renal capsule and projecting outward are distinguished from parenchymal cysts **(Fig. 48.2)**, and parapelvic and pelvic cysts. These latter cysts can be mistaken for obstruction and dilation of the renal pelvis **(31)** (see pp. 52 and 63). The examiner should note the diameter of the cyst and its location (upper or lower pole; or upper, middle, or lower third of the kidney) and carefully examine its immediate vicinity for any signs of a tumorous mass. Some malignant renal tumors contain cystic components that may be significantly more conspicuous than the actual solid component of the tumor.

Isolated renal cysts are of no clinical significance and require only long-term follow-up. In contrast, the adult form of familial polycystic disease **(Fig. 48.3)** can produce multiple cysts with progressive growth in middle age. These cysts can reach a considerable size.

Polycystic degeneration leads to kidney failure in early adulthood as a result of displacement and thinning of the renal parenchyma. These patients eventually require dialysis.

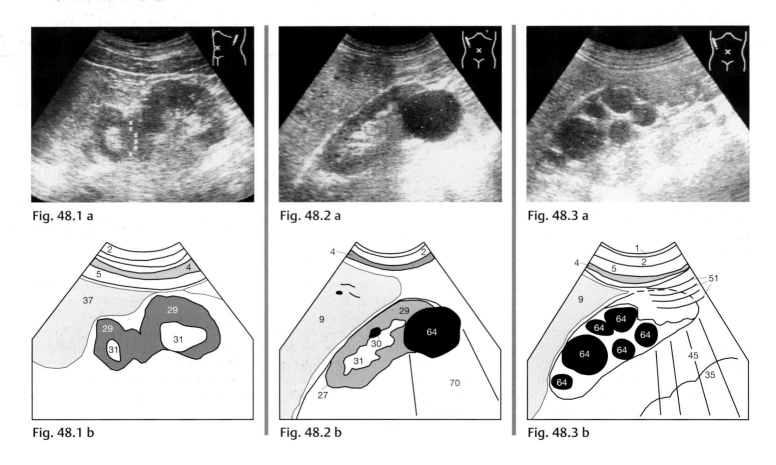

Fig. 48.1 a

Fig. 48.2 a

Fig. 48.3 a

Fig. 48.1 b

Fig. 48.2 b

Fig. 48.3 b

The next two pages present the crucial morphologic characteristics in newborns and children that differ from findings in adults.

Kidneys in Newborns

Before examining the kidneys in the prone newborn (**Fig. 49.1a**), one should first examine the bladder with the patient supine as it can only be evaluated when full and newborns often void during the examination. After this, the patient is positioned prone and posteroanterior scans of both kidneys are performed in the longitudinal plane (**Fig. 49.1**) and transverse plane (**Fig. 49.2**) using a 5.0–7.5 MHz linear transducer. Anteroposterior transhepatic scanning (see p. 47) or lateroposterior examination with the patient in the lateral decubitus position is more suitable only in older infants. Lower center frequencies of 3.5–3.75 MHz are preferred in older children. Reference values of childrens' kidneys are defined in percentiles depending on childrens' body height. A summary may be found on page 53.

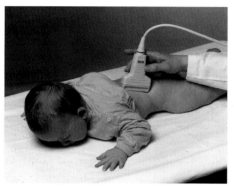

Fig. 49.1 a

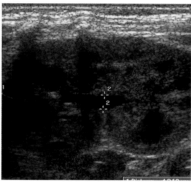

Fig. 49.1 b

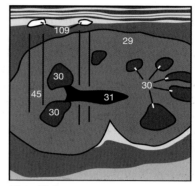

Fig. 49.1 c

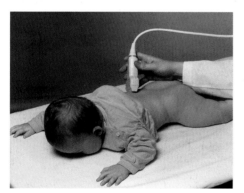

Fig. 49.2 a

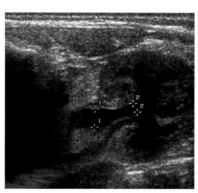

Fig. 49.2 b

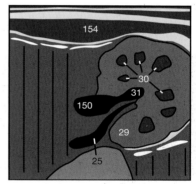

Fig. 49.2 c

Typical Variants in Newborns

Compared with adults, the kidney in newborns shows a more hyperechoic outer parenchyma (**29**) with sharper contrast to the hypoechoic medullary pyramids (**30**). The triangular shape of the medullary pyramids is therefore more sharply defined in newborns than in adults, whose pyramids appear more rounded.

Many neonatal kidneys also show residual fetal lobulation and gradually assume an increasingly smooth oval contour only later in infancy. The hyperechoic central renal caliceal system (**31**) initially appears as a thin line in newborns and only increases gradually in width during infancy. This is due to the increasing deposition of fat between blood vessels and calices.

As a result the anechoic renal pelvis is more conspicuous in a newborn. It can measure up to 5 mm in width in the absence of any urinary obstruction (see p. 54).

The "dromedary hump," a bulge in the left lateral renal cortex opposite the lower pole of the spleen, is also typical of the shape of the kidney in younger children and usually disappears as the organ grows. Hyperplastic columns of Bertin can traverse the hyperechoic pelvic region as hypoechoic parenchymal bridges, mimicking renal duplication (see **Fig. 48.1**). Neither finding has a mass effect, and neither should be confused with a renal tumor.

Diffusely Increased Echogenicity

Diffusely increased echogenicity in the renal parenchyma in newborns is regarded as normal (see previous page). Yet even in later infancy it is a sign of parenchymal damage (**Fig. 50.1**). Findings then include renal parenchyma (**29**) that appears isoechoic or hyperechoic to the liver (**9**) and particularly to the medullary pyramids (**30**).

Aside from glomerulonephritis, possible causes include diffuse leukemic infiltration and medication-induced damage such as can occur secondary to multiple chemotherapy (**Fig. 50.2**), shown here with nascent obstruction in the renal pelvis (**31**).

Diffusely increased echogenicity in the kidney should invariably prompt the examiner to search for pleural effusion (see **Fig. 39.3**) and ascites in the true pelvis (**Fig. 50.3**). In the presence of proteinuria and hypoproteinemia, such findings suggest nephrotic syndrome. The example in **Fig. 50.3** was intentionally selected to emphasize the risk of misinterpretation when the examination is performed after voiding. The bladder (**38**) is nearly empty after voiding, so that the ascites (**68**) adjacent to the small uterus (**39**) could easily be mistaken for the bladder.

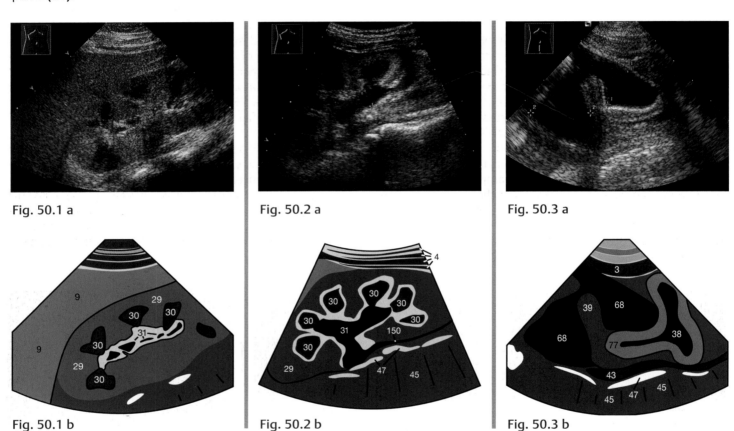

Fig. 50.1 a

Fig. 50.2 a

Fig. 50.3 a

Fig. 50.1 b

Fig. 50.2 b

Fig. 50.3 b

Nephrocalcinosis

The deposition of crystals that occurs in nephrocalcinosis initially creates a hyperechoic rim around the medullary pyramids, later extending to the caliceal apices or diffusely throughout the pyramids. This inverts the contrast between these structures, with hyperechoic medullary pyramids and a relatively hypoechoic parenchymal rim. The calcifications initially show no acoustic shadowing.

Possible causes include tubular acidosis, urate nephropathy with massive cell destruction in the setting of chemotherapy, vitamin D overdose, and therapy with ACTH or furosemide. The picture of diffusely hyperechoic medullary pyramids resembles that in a dehydrated newborn with protein precipitation. These deposits of Tamm–Horsfall protein are reversible within a few days when the newborn is rehydrated.

Nephritis

The kidney reacts to various causes of inflammation with a relatively uniform morphologic picture. The kidney can appear normal in acute pyelonephritis or where inflammation is limited to the glomeruli. However, it later increases in size due to edema. Interstitial infiltration also increases the echogenicity of the parenchyma (29). This increases its contrast against the hypoechoic medullary pyramids (30 in Fig. 51.3) and gives the medullary pyramids a "punched out" appearance. The parenchyma of the inflamed, infiltrated kidney appears significantly more hyperechoic (Fig. 51.3) compared with the adjacent spleen or liver (9) than it normally does (see Fig. 48.3).

Unfortunately, the increased echogenicity of the renal parenchyma does not allow any conclusions about the cause of the inflammation. The same phenomenon occurs with interstitial nephritis, chronic glomerulonephritis, diabetic nephropathy, renal amyloidosis (autoimmune infiltration), and urate nephropathy. This latter form results from an elevated serum uric acid concentration in gout or increased tissue destruction. Ultrasound does not make any significant contribution to a differential diagnosis among the various causes of inflammation. However, it is useful for following up nephritis during therapy and for excluding additional complications. Doppler sonography can be used to determine the resistance index (a measure of renal perfusion), which can provide valuable information about the course of infiltration or the onset of acute rejection in transplanted kidneys. Ultrasound-guided needle biopsy can obtain renal tissue for histologic evaluation.

In acute nephritis, the parenchyma can be diffusely hypoechoic and widened, and the border between the parenchyma and renal pelvis can appear indistinct or blurred. In normal kidneys it is invariably sharply demarcated.

Renal Degeneration

With increasing age slow, progressive narrowing of the parenchyma may be observed. This narrowing is physiologic (see p. 47), but increased parenchymal atrophy (Fig. 51.1) also occurs secondary to repeated inflammation or in the setting of high-grade renal artery stenosis. Reduced perfusion can involve the entire kidney or circumscribed infarcts can occur, as is often the case in embolic disorders (see Fig. 56.3). In end-stage disease, narrowing of the parenchyma (29) can be so pronounced that it is barely visualized (Fig. 51.2). This imaging example of a shrunken kidney shows the most common associated findings of degenerative calcifications (53) or calculi (49) that are visualized indirectly because of their acoustic shadows (45). Shrunken kidneys can be so small that ultrasound scans fail to detect them.

Loss of function in a kidney can be fully compensated by the contralateral kidney, which shows compensatory hypertrophy. When a shrunken kidney is detected, one should first determine the parenchyma to pelvis index (see p. 47). A normal index suggests congenital renal hypoplasia. Usually the combination of examination of the contralateral kidney and color duplex ultrasound evaluation of renal perfusion can establish a diagnosis.

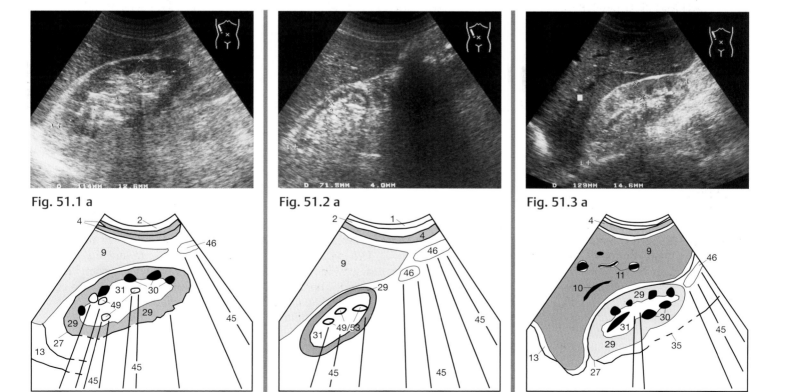

Fig. 51.1 a

Fig. 51.2 a

Fig. 51.3 a

Fig. 51.1 b

Fig. 51.2 b

Fig. 51.3 b

Normally, the collecting system appears as a very hyperechoic central complex traversed only by narrow hypoechoic lines corresponding to small blood vessels or parts of the collecting system. As diuresis increases after intake of a large amount of fluid, the hypoechoic collecting system (87) within the pelvic complex (31) can appear more pronounced than usual (Fig. 52.1). The developmental variant of an extrarenal pelvis has a similar appearance. The dilation present in both physiologic conditions does not involve the caliceal neck.

Three degrees of urinary obstruction are distinguished in adults. In first-degree obstruction, the renal sinus (87) is dilated but, as in the variants mentioned above, the dilation does not involve caliceal necks (Fig. 52.2). The thickness of the parenchyma is normal. In second-degree urinary obstruction, the caliceal necks and calices are thickened as well (Fig. 52.3). Additionally, beginning parenchymal thinning may also be detectable. Third-degree urinary obstruction is characterized by extensive pressure atrophy of the renal parenchyma as well.

Ultrasound examination can only demonstrate a few of the possible causes of urinary obstruction. A ureteral stone is generally only visualized proximally at the ureteropelvic junction or distally at the ureterovesical junction. The mid-ureter is usually obscured by overlying intestinal air. An exception is seen in Fig. 52.4, which shows a stone (49) in the ureter (150).

Rare causes of ureteral obstruction are tumors of the bladder or uterus and retroperitoneal fibrosis, either secondary to radiation therapy or as an idiopathic disorder (Ormond disease). Retroperitoneal lymph node conglomerates can cause ureteral compression. Latent obstruction can be caused by an atonic ureter in pregnancy, infections, and incomplete emptying of the bladder (neurogenic or in advanced prostatic hypertrophy, see p. 75). In these cases, the post-void residual bladder volume (see p. 59) is measured.

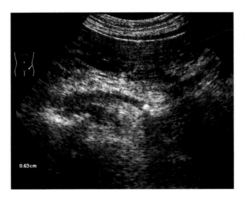

Fig. 52.4 a

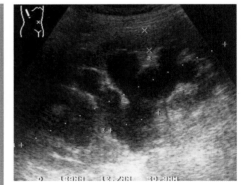

Fig. 52.4 b

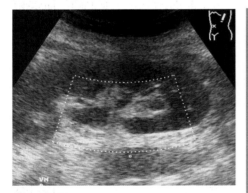

Fig. 52.1 a

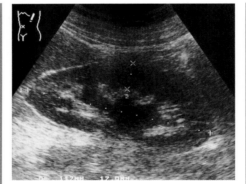

Fig. 52.2 a

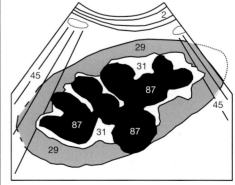

Fig. 52.3 a

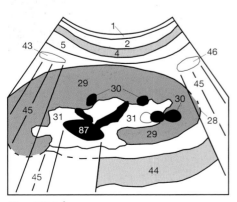

Fig. 52.1 b

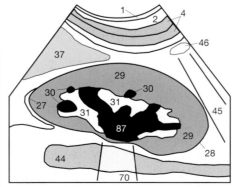

Fig. 52.2 b

Fig. 52.3 b

Not every hypoechoic dilation of the renal pelvis (31) indicates a urinary obstruction. The developmental variant of an extrarenal pelvis was already mentioned on the preceding page.

The renal hilum can also show prominent blood vessels (25 in Fig. 53.1) that can be traced into the hypoechoic medullary pyramids (30) and mistaken for structures of the collecting system. These vessels generally appear rather delicate, and do not show the characteristic clubbing of hypoechoic structures seen in urinary obstruction (Fig. 52.2). The differential diagnosis can be made quickly by determining the flow with color-coded duplex sonography. With an adequate setting, blood flow is displayed as color while the static or only slowly flowing urine remains anechoic (= black). Differentiating

urinary obstruction (87) from parapelvic or pelvic cysts (64) is more difficult (Fig. 53.2), particularly if both conditions are present. Urinary obstruction in children is discussed on pp. 54 and 55.

Alternative Methods

Where ultrasound examination is unable to determine the nature of a urinary obstruction, supplementary noninvasive modalities such as computed tomography (CT, Fig. 53.3) or an intravenous urogram (Fig. 53.4) can be used. Either method can quantify the dilation of both the pelvicaliceal system (⇩) and the ureter (⬈). Figures 53.3 and 53.4 show the same patient, who has caliceal dilation that is more severe on the left than on the right, and obstructive ureteral dilation.

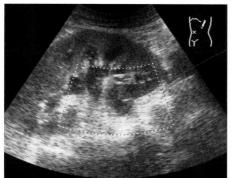

Fig. 53.1 a

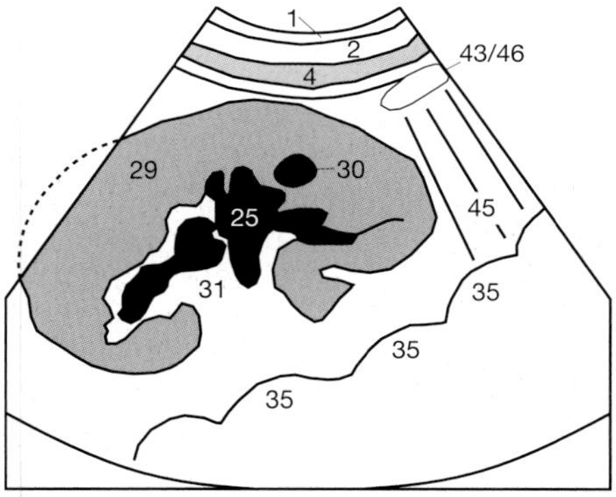

Fig. 53.2a

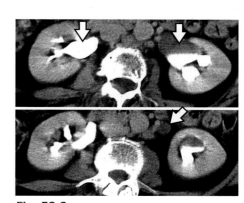

Fig. 53.3

Fig. 53.1 b

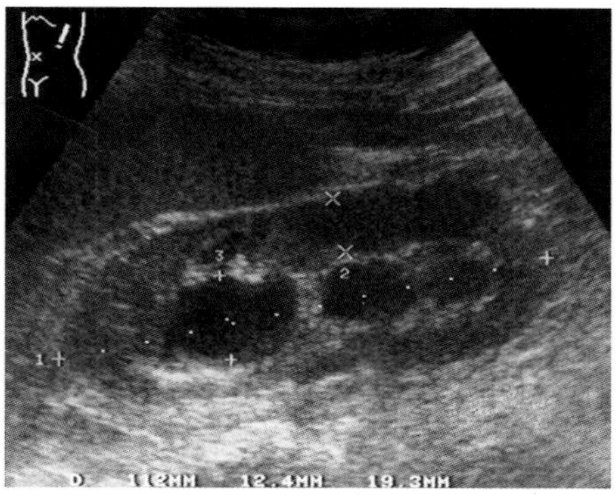

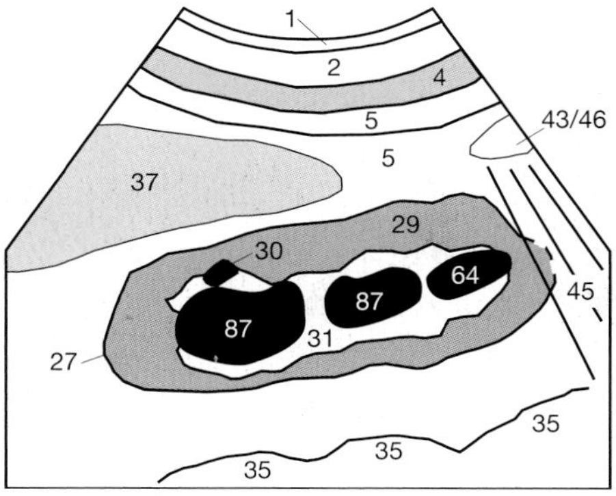

Fig. 53.2 b

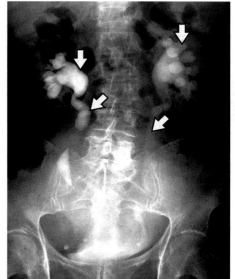

Fig. 53.4

Normal Values of the kidneys in pediatrics
(For a German population, according to Dinkel E. et al.: Kidney Size in Childhood, Pediatr Radiol (15): 38–43)

Body size (cm)	$\overline{m}$ - 2 SD	$\overline{m}$	$\overline{m}$ + 2 SD
Newborns	3.40	4.16	4.92
< 55	3.00	4.35	5.70
55 – 70	3.60	5.00	6.40
71 – 85	4.50	5.90	7.30
86 – 100	5.30	6.60	7.90
101 – 110	5.85	7.10	8.35
111 – 120	6.35	7.65	8.95
121 – 130	6.90	8.20	9.50
131 – 140	7.40	8.70	10.00
141 – 150	7.90	9.25	10.60
> 150	8.60	9.95	11.30

P

When the initial ultrasound screening examination of a newborn is performed, it is crucial to detect any stenosis of the ureteropelvic or ureterovesical junction or any vesicoureteral reflux with secondary obstruction so as to avoid any subsequent damage to the kidneys.

Remember that the delicate anechoic renal pelvis (31) can be up to 5 mm wide in newborns (Fig. 54.1) in the absence of any urinary obstruction. Where the renal pelvis measures between 5 and 10 mm in width (Fig. 54.2), follow-up examinations at short intervals are indicated to clarify whether findings represent a congenital extrarenal pelvis or a pathologic progressive dilation of the collecting system. Only a renal pelvis exceeding 10 mm in width (Fig. 54.3), clubbed calices (149), and a dilated ureter (150) are indications for an immediate diagnostic workup (Fig. 54.3). A voiding cystourethrogram is generally obtained (see next page).

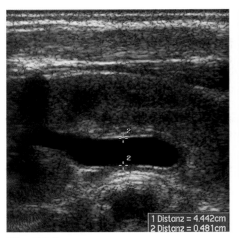

Fig. 54.1 a

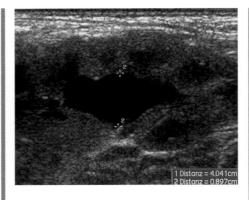

Fig. 54.2 a

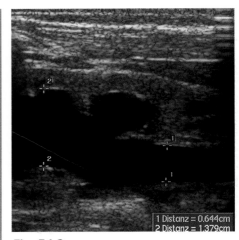

Fig. 54.3 a

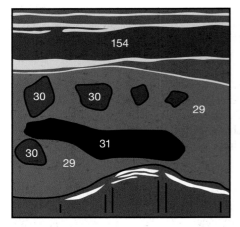

Fig. 54.1 b

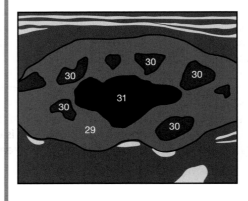

Fig. 54.2 b

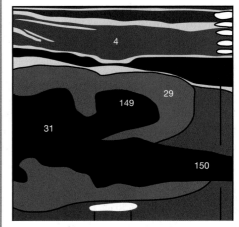

Fig. 54.3 b

Where both the renal pelvis (31) and the ureter (150) are dilated as in Fig. 54.3, a ureteropelvic stenosis can be reliably excluded as the cause of the urinary obstruction. However, isolated dilation of the renal pelvis with or without caliceal clubbing should be further evaluated with a voiding cystourethrogram or intravenous urogram to exclude vesicoureteral reflux or stenosis of the ureteropelvic junction. The example in Fig. 54.3 shows a thinned parenchymal cortex due to urinary obstruction. Immediate diagnostic workup is indicated and possibly decompression as well.

Width of the renal pelvis in newborns:	
Normal	< 5 mm
Follow-up indicated	5–10 mm
Possible pathologic dilation	> 10 mm

Possible Sequelae of Urinary Obstruction

When urinary obstruction is not detected early, it can lead to thinning of the parenchyma (**29** in **Fig. 55.1**) and gradually progress to a shrunken kidney (see **Fig. 51.2**) with corresponding loss of renal function. Chronic urinary tract infections or metabolic disorders can also induce crystalline deposits (➘) in the dilated calices of the pelvicaliceal system (**Fig. 55.2**).

Grades of Reflux in Children	
Grade I	Reflux into distal ureter
Grade II	Reflux into pelvicaliceal system
Grade III	Additional beginning ureteral dilation and caliceal clubbing
Grade IV	Increasing ureteral dilation and caliceal clubbing
Grade V	Pronounced ureteral dilation and beginning parenchymal thinning

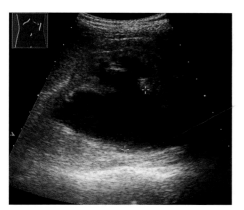

Fig. 55.1 a

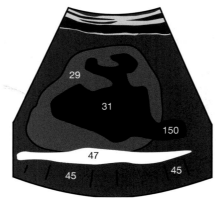

Fig. 55.1 b

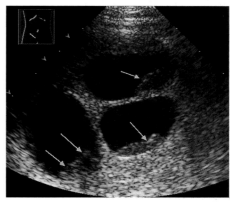

Fig. 55.2

Voiding Cystourethrogram

A voiding cystourethrogram (micturating cystourethrogram, MCU) excludes or confirms vesicoureteral reflux and should be performed in patients with recurrent urinary tract infections or urinary obstruction in the infection-free interval after antibiotic therapy. Normally (**Fig. 55.3**), the full bladder shows no retrograde reflux into the ureter (◄►) even during voiding through the urethra (➡). The images are obtained in a slightly oblique projection to avoid misinterpreting the adjacent cortex of the ilium (imaged end on) as grade I reflux (into distal ureter only). Reflux into the collecting system (◄) is referred to as grade II reflux (**Fig. 55.4**). Grade III is characterized by extensive dilation of the ureter and beginning clubbing of the calices.

Grade IV reflux in children is characterized by increasing caliceal clubbing and ureteral dilation; grade V refers to cases where parenchymal thinning is also present (see table). The chronic end stage is characterized by tortuosity of the entire dilated ureter as seen in **Fig. 55.5**.

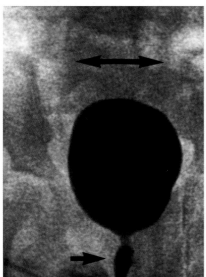

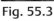

Fig. 55.3

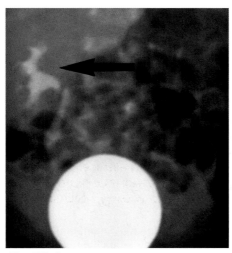

Fig. 55.4

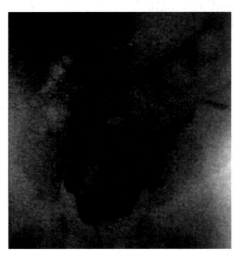

Fig. 55.5

Detecting stones in the kidney (nephrolithiasis) is more difficult than detecting stones in the gallbladder (see p. 44) because the hyperechoic stones (49) often lie within the equally hyperechoic renal pelvis (31 in **Fig. 56.1**) and therefore are not contrasted against relatively hypoechoic fluid. Stones in an obstructed renal sinus are a notable exception as the contrast is greater here. The examiner must be particularly alert to acoustic shadows (45) caused by kidney stones or calcifications. **Fig. 56.2** shows an example of extensive renal calcifications (49) in a patient with hyperparathyroidism and a markedly elevated serum calcium level.

Depending on its composition, a kidney stone (49) can transmit sound without attenuation (**Fig. 56.1**) or be so reflective that only its proximal surface is visualized as hyperechoic dome (**Fig. 56.2**). The differential diagnosis includes arcuate arteries between the renal cortex and the medullary pyramids (bright echoes without acoustic shadows), vascular calcifications in diabetic patients, and calcified scarring secondary to renal tuberculosis. Papillary calcifications secondary to phenacetin abuse are a less common cause.

Large staghorn calculi are difficult to diagnose if there is only weak distal acoustic shadowing because the large calculus can easily be mistaken for the hyperechoic renal pelvis.

Renal concrements can dislodge and migrate into the ureter (**Fig. 52.4**). Depending on their size, they can pass into the bladder unnoticed or produce coliclike symptoms. They can also become lodged in the ureter and cause acute obstruction. In addition to detecting urinary obstruction, ultrasound can exclude other causes of pain, such as pancreatitis, colitis, and free fluid in the pouch of Douglas (see p. 60).

Renal Infarcts

Circumscribed renal infarcts (71) have been observed as a result of renal emboli from an aortic aneurysm (see p. 23) or renal artery stenosis. These infarcts conform to arterial territories and are broad-based at the renal surface and tapered toward the renal hilum. The result is a triangular defect (**Fig. 56.3**) in the parenchyma (29), which in the late stage progresses to a hyperechoic scar. The location and typical shape of these hyperechoic scars can help distinguish them from kidney stones or renal tumors.

In addition to digital subtraction angiography (DSA), noninvasive color-coded duplex sonography is useful for detecting renal artery stenosis. Visualizing and evaluating small accessory renal arteries is especially difficult. They can arise from the aorta in the immediate vicinity of the main renal artery, or they can arise from the aorta farther from it as upper or lower "polar arteries." In rare cases, they can also arise from the common iliac artery.

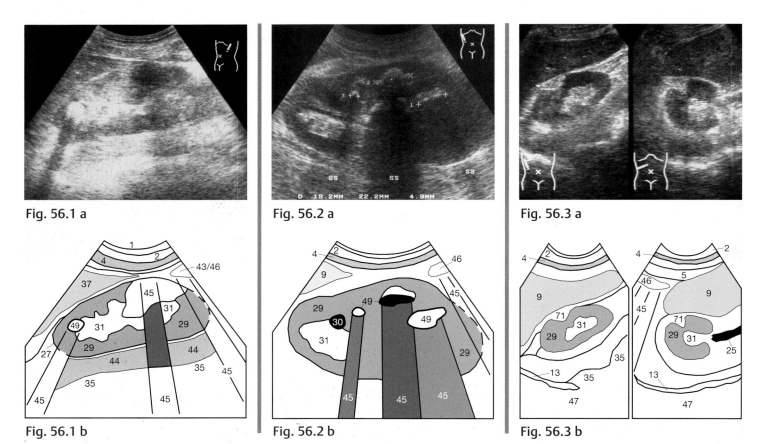

Fig. 56.1 a

Fig. 56.2 a

Fig. 56.3 a

Fig. 56.1 b

Fig. 56.2 b

Fig. 56.3 b

Solid renal tumors are distinguished from fluid-filled cysts by internal echoes and only weak or absent distal acoustic enhancement.

Benign Renal Tumors

Solid benign renal tumors (fibromas, adenomas, and hemangiomas) are altogether rare and show an inhomogeneous morphology on ultrasound images. Only the angiomyolipoma – a benign mixed tumor comprising vessels, muscular tissue, and fat – has a characteristic appearance in its early stage that clearly distinguishes it from a malignant process. A small angiomyolipoma **(72)** is similarly hyperechoic and sharply demarcated **(Fig. 57.1)** as the renal pelvis **(31)**. Its sonographic morphology resembles that of a hepatic hemangioma **(Figs. 39.2** and **39.3)**. Angiomy lipomas only become inhomogeneous as their size increases; they then become difficult to differentiate from malignant tumors.

Malignant Renal Tumors

Small renal cell carcinomas **(54)** are often isoechoic to the rest of the renal parenchyma **(29)**. Only as their growth progresses do they become more inhomogeneous and create a bulge in the contour of the kidney **(Fig. 57.2)**. If a carcinoma has been detected, both renal veins and the inferior vena cava must be carefully examined for tumor tissue to exclude vascular invasion. Renal carcinomas occasionally develop tumorous extensions into these vessels and occur bilaterally in up to 5% of all cases. If the tumor penetrates the renal capsule and infiltrates the surrounding tissue, the kidney can lose its normal mobility with respiration (see p. 47). Some malignant renal tumors can also contain cystic components. Therefore it is important to look for solid masses in the vicinity of what appear to be benign renal cysts.

Adrenal Tumors

The left adrenal gland lies anteromedial (not superior) to the upper pole of the left kidney. The right adrenal gland usually lies slightly superior to the upper pole of the right kidney and posterior to the inferior vena cava. In adults, both adrenal glands are largely obscured by the perirenal fat. This is not the case with the adrenal glands in newborns (see p. 58).

Hormone-producing adrenal tumors such as adenomas in aldosteronism (Conn syndrome) or hyperplasia in the setting of Cushing syndrome are generally too small to be detectable on ultrasound. Clinically apparent pheochromocytomas are the only such lesions that can usually be detected on ultrasound. By the time symptoms appear, these lesions will often have attained a size of several centimeters so that 90% of them are detectable. When in doubt, order a supplementary CT scan.

Ultrasound is more helpful in detecting adrenal metastases **(54)**, which usually appear as hypoechoic masses **(Fig. 57.3)** between the upper pole of the kidney and the spleen **(37)** or inferior margin of the liver, respectively. These metastases must be differentiated from superficial renal cysts. Because the adrenal glands are richly vascularized, hematogenous spread of metastases from carcinomas of the lung, breast and kidney is common. The echogenicity of a suprarenal mass neither allows a conclusion as to whether it is benign or malignant, nor does it differentiate the mass from a neurinoma arising from the sympathetic chain.

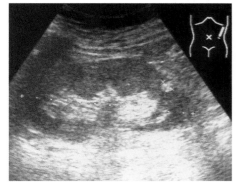

Fig. 57.1 a

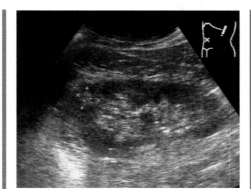

Fig. 57.2 a

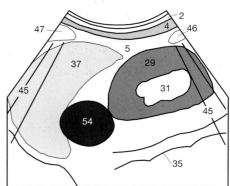

Fig. 57.3 a

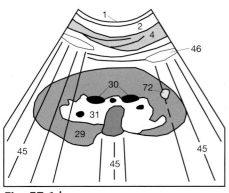

Fig. 57.1 b

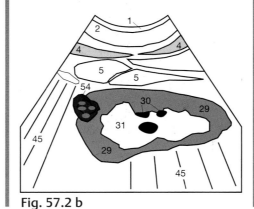

Fig. 57.2 b

Fig. 57.3 b

Benign Renal Tumors

Aside from fibromas in neurofibromatosis (Recklinghausen disease), benign masses in the pediatric kidney include angiomyolipomas, which occur in combination with Bourneville–Pringle disease (tuberous sclerosis) and resemble adult angiomyolipomas (**Fig. 57.1**).

Nephroblastoma

The nephroblastoma (**54**) is the most common mass encountered in children (**Figs. 58.1** and **58.2**). Also known as Wilms tumor, it leads to complete destruction of the normal renal anatomy and frequently exhibits an inhomogeneous hyperechoic internal structure and impairs urinary drainage from the remaining parenchyma (**29**) as in **Fig. 58.3**. It is important to examine the contralateral kidney to exclude bilateral involvement, which is observed in up to 10% of all cases.

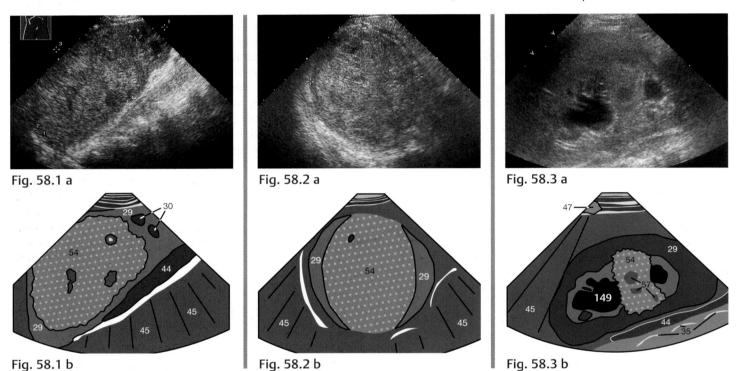

Fig. 58.1 a   Fig. 58.2 a   Fig. 58.3 a

Fig. 58.1 b   Fig. 58.2 b   Fig. 58.3 b

Lymphomatous Infiltration and Metastases

Malignant infiltration of the kidneys from lymphomas or metastatic disease is less common. The difference in echogenicity between involved areas and normal renal parenchyma (**29**) may not be very conspicuous (**Fig. 58.3**), and such lesions are often identifiable only by central necrosis (**57**) or associated urinary obstruction in adjacent caliceal groups (**149**).

Adrenal Gland

In newborns and preterm neonates, the hypoechoic adrenal cortex can invariably be distinguished from the hyperechoic medulla (**155** in **Fig. 58.4**). On a posteroanterior scan, the adrenal gland typically appears as a Y shape superolateral to the upper pole of the kidney. This difference in echogenicity disappears during infancy and adult adrenal glands are barely distinguishable from perirenal fat (see **Fig. 51.1**).

In newborns, bleeding in the adrenal glands is usually visualized as a hypoechoic area ( ) at the upper pole of the kidney (**Fig. 58.5**). If this finding is indeed a hematoma, it should measurably decrease in size within a month. If its size is unchanged, laboratory tests or MRI must be performed to exclude a cystic neuroblastoma. Adenomas of the adrenal gland are less common. Because of their small size they are often detectable only on noncontrasted high-resolution CT densitometry studies.

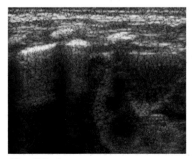 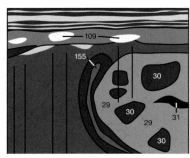 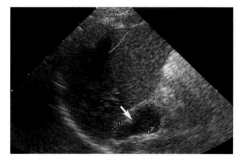

Fig. 58.4 a   Fig. 58.4 b   Fig. 58.5

Examination Technique

The bladder is systematically scanned in suprapubic transverse (**Fig. 59.1a**) and sagittal (**Fig.59.1b**) planes. The examiner must perform the scan slowly enough to detect any suspicious wall thickening or intraluminal masses. Including the adjacent lateral perivesical tissue in the scan has proven effective. Wherever possible, the examination should be performed with the patient's bladder maximally filled after drinking a large amount of clear liquid and before voiding or, in catheterized patients, after clamping the indwelling catheter. This will better visualize the bladder wall. Examining the empty bladder after the patient has voided has no diagnostic value.

On a typical transverse image (**Fig. 59.2**), the normal bladder (38) lies posterior to the two rectus abdominis muscles (3) and cranial and anterior to the rectum (43). When filled to capacity, the bladder exhibits the shape of a rectangle with rounded corners. In the sagittal plane (**Fig. 59.3**), the bladder appears more triangular. The prostate gland (42) or vagina is visualized caudal to the bladder (see **Figs. 75.2** and **77.1**).

Determining Post-voiding Residual Bladder Volume

Where neurogenic dysfunction or obstruction due to hypertrophy of the prostate gland (see p. 75) is suspected, the bladder volume should be calculated to determine the post-voiding residual bladder volume. The maximum transverse diameter (**Fig. 59.2b**) is determined on the transverse

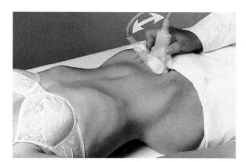

Fig. 59.1 a

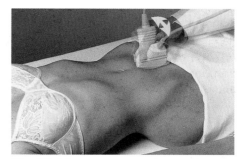

Fig. 59.1 b

image and the maximum craniocaudal diameter on the sagittal image (the horizontal dotted line in **Fig. 59.3b**). To obtain a suitable sagittal scan, it will often be necessary to tilt the transducer caudally as shown in **Fig. 59.3a** to work around the acoustic shadow (45) of the pubic bone (48). The maximum anteroposterior diameter (vertically dotted line on both images) must then be determined in one of the two planes.

The post-voiding residual bladder volume is then calculated in milliliters according to the simplified volume formula as the product of the three diameters multiplied by 0.5. Even though a post-voiding residual bladder volume up to 100 mL has been described as physiologic in the literature, one should consider an outlet obstruction wherever the post-voiding residual bladder volume exceeds 50 mL.

Determining Bladder Volume
Bladder volume = A x B x C x 0.5

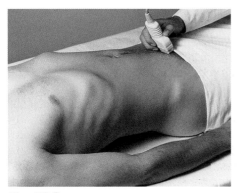

Fig. 59.2 a

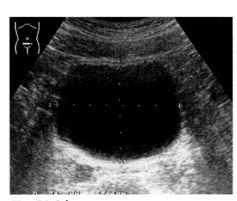

Fig. 59.2 b

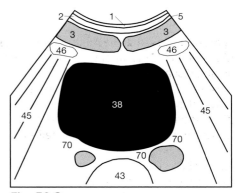

Fig. 59.2 c

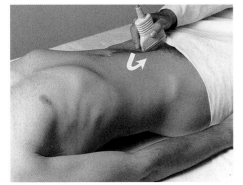

Fig. 59.3 a

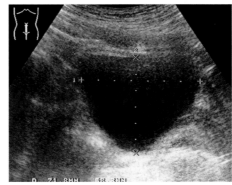

Fig. 59.3 b

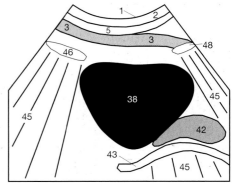

Fig. 59.3 c

In patients with an indwelling catheter (76) the bladder (38) is usually collapsed, effectively preventing reliable evaluation. Therefore the catheter should be clamped some time prior to the examination (remember to do this!) to fill the urinary bladder. Cystitis (**Fig. 60.2**) can be diagnosed in an empty bladder only in the presence of an advanced edema of the bladder wall (77). Wall thickness in a distended (filled) bladder should not exceed 4 mm. After voiding, even the normal bladder wall is irregular and up to 8 mm thick, potentially masking mural polyps or circumscribed tumors.

Wall Thickening

Diffuse wall thickening involving the entire circumference is usually due to edema in the setting of cystitis. A circumscribed area of wall thickening is more suggestive of a tumor adherent to the wall. The differential diagnosis in males must consider a trabeculated bladder, which can occur in response to a bladder outlet obstruction in prostatic hypertrophy. When in doubt, transrectal or (in females) transvaginal ultrasound at higher frequencies or CT studies can provide more information.

Internal Echoes and Sedimentation

Even the healthy bladder is never entirely anechoic (= black). Reverberation artifacts (51a) induced by the anterior abdominal wall (**Fig. 60.3**) are usually projected into the lumen of the bladder (38) near the transducer. Section thickness artifacts (51b) are often observed in the posterior bladder distal to the transducer. These are caused by the oblique course of the bladder wall relative to the sound beam and can mimic intraluminal matter (see p. 16). These artifacts must be differentiated from actual sediments of crystals, small blood clots

(52), or calculi (49) along the bladder floor (**Fig. 60.3**). Sediment can be mobilized by rapidly varying the pressure applied to the transducer (be careful with a full bladder ...). This maneuver will naturally fail to separate a mural tumor from the bladder wall.

Ureteral Peristalsis

Incidental findings occasionally include signs of inflow into the bladder from the ureteral ostia due to propulsive ureteral peristalsis. In infants one must also exclude an ureterocele (see **Fig. 61.4**).

Free Fluid

In any abdominal trauma, it is essential to confirm or exclude free fluid (68) in the abdomen. **Fig. 60.4** shows free fluid (68) in its typical location in the pouch of Douglas posterior to the uterus (39), such as can occur in acute intra-abdominal bleeding.

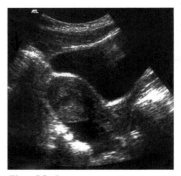

Fig. 60.4 a

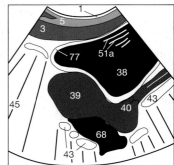

Fig. 60.4 b

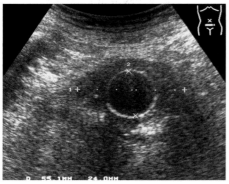

Fig. 60.1 a

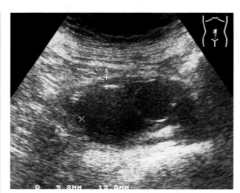

Fig. 60.2 a

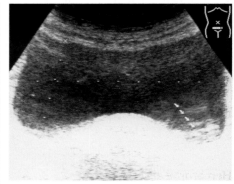

Fig. 60.3 a

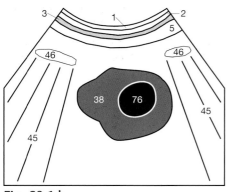

Fig. 60.1 b

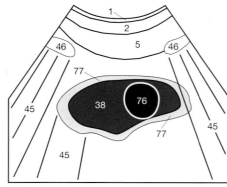

Fig. 60.2 b

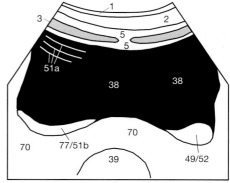

Fig. 60.3 b

Patent Urachus

In the newborn, the bladder is best examined in longitudinal and transverse suprapubic planes (Fig. 61.1a) as long as it is still filled (this means at the beginning of the examination!). Particular attention should be paid to the roof of the bladder (Fig. 61.1b) to avoid missing a patent urachus. This will appear as a hypoechoic channel (↖) along the anterior abdominal wall between the umbilicus (↑) and the roof of the bladder (Fig. 61.2).

Fig. 61.1 a

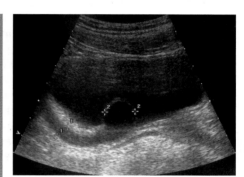

Fig. 61.1 b

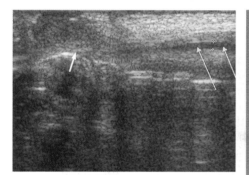

Fig. 61.2 a

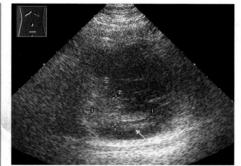

Fig. 61.3 a

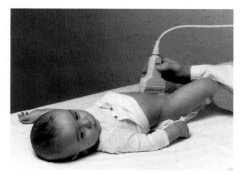

Fig. 61.4 a

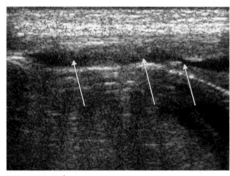

Fig. 61.2 b

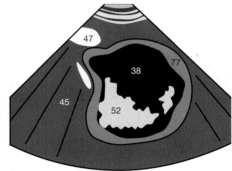

Fig. 61.3 b

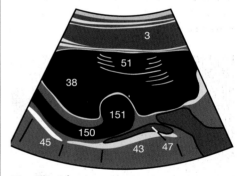

Fig. 61.4 b

Hematoma and Cystitis

In children, the most common masses in the urinary bladder (38) are blood clots (52), which usually occur in the setting of hemorrhagic cystitis (Fig. 61.3). This child received chemotherapy in preparation for a bone marrow transplant. As in adults (Fig. 60.2), cystitis manifests itself as wall thickening (77).

Ureterocele

In infants presenting with urinary obstruction, one must exclude a uterocele (151) in addition to ureteral obstruction at the ureteropelvic or ureterovesical junction. An ureterocele can project into the bladder lumen as a thin membranous structure (Fig. 61.4) that can change size and shape depending on the level of filling. This image also shows a dilated distal ureter (150).

P

Renal transplants are placed in the right or left iliac fossa and connected to the iliac vessels. They are systematically scanned in two planes **(Fig. 62.1)** like native kidneys. The only difference is that the transducer must be placed over the lateral lower abdomen with the patient supine. Because of the superficial position of the renal transplant, there is typically no interposed intestinal gas. This position greatly facilitates the ultrasound follow-up examination.

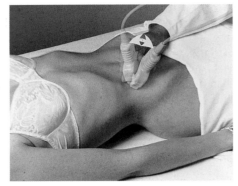

Fig. 62.1 a

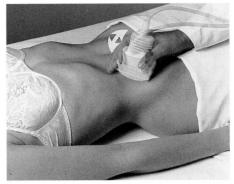

Fig. 62.1 b

Normal Appearance of Renal Transplants

A normal transplanted kidney can show a volume increase of up to 20%, which is usually permanent. The parenchyma **(29)** appears wider **(Fig. 62.2)** than in native kidneys. Its echogenicity may be greater, increasing the contrast to the medullary pyramids **(30)** in comparison with native kidneys. Ultrasound follow-up studies at close intervals are initially indicated to exclude progressive inflammatory infiltration. A prominent fluid-filled renal pelvis or grade I urinary obstruction (see **Figs. 52.1** and **52.2**) is often observed, but without a functional impairment of the transplant that would justify intervention. The obstruction is best documented on the transverse image **(Fig. 62.3)** and carefully measured to avoid missing progressive obstruction that may require therapeutic intervention.

Early Detection of Rejection

The renal transplant should be further evaluated for sharp demarcation against surrounding tissues and for a sharply demarcated border between the parenchyma **(29)** and renal pelvis **(31)**. Blurring of the border between parenchyma and renal pelvis or an increase in volume since the previous examination can be warning signs of beginning rejection.

Therefore, longitudinal and transverse diameters are measured and documented to allow a valid comparison with subsequent studies (see p. 63). Doppler sonography is then used to determine the resistance index of the vessels in the transplant. This is an important indicator of the onset of acute rejection. In the absence of rejection, both the dosage of immunosuppressives and the frequency of follow-up examinations can be reduced over time.

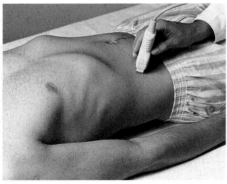

Fig. 62.2 a

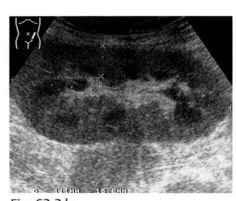

Fig. 62.2 b

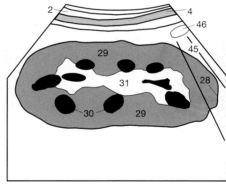

Fig. 62.2 c

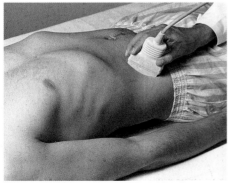

Fig. 62.3 a

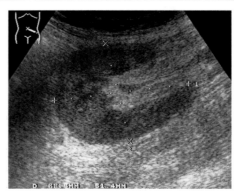

Fig. 62.3 b

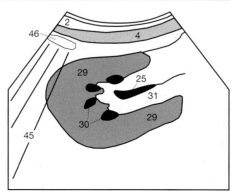

Fig. 62.3 c

To obtain an accurate size measurement, first scan the transplant in the longitudinal plane (**Fig. 63.1b**) until you have visualized its maximum length. The diagram in **Fig. 63.1a** illustrates how choosing an imaging plane too far lateral (dotted line) would falsify the length measurement by making the kidney appear too short. The transducer must be tilted in the direction of the straight black arrows to obtain an accurate longitudinal length measurement (d_L).

Then the transducer is rotated slightly (**Fig. 63.1c**) to make sure that the kidney has not been visualized obliquely as indicated by the second dotted black line in **Fig. 63.1a**. Any such angulation must be eliminated by rotating the transducer in the direction of the curved arrow. The purpose of this two-step manipulation of the transducer is to avoid errors that might cause you to document a foreshortened length. Such a measurement error could lead to subsequent misdiagnosis because what appears to be increased volume on follow-up images would suggest a rejection reaction.

Lymphocele

A postoperative lymphocele (**73**) can develop as a complication of transplant surgery (**Fig. 63.2**). Lymphoceles usually occur between the lower pole of the transplanted kidney (**29**) and the bladder (**38**), although they are also observed elsewhere in the vicinity of the transplant. Not every lymphocele is an indication for intervention. Small lymphoceles often resolve spontaneously. Large lymphoceles can occasionally be initially mistaken for the bladder.

Urinary Obstruction

Urinary obstruction (**87**) is also a common postoperative complication that can result from reimplantation of the ureter. Depending on its severity, it can require temporary placement of a catheter (**59**) to ensure drainage (**Figs. 63.3** and **63.4**) so as to prevent damage to the parenchyma (**29**) of the transplant.

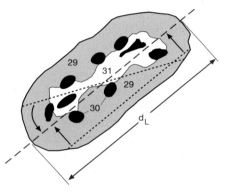

Fig. 63.1 a

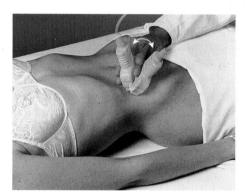

Fig. 63.1 b

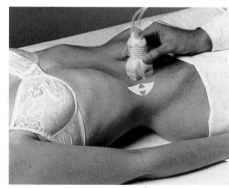

Fig. 63.1 c

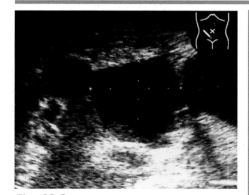

Fig. 63.2 a

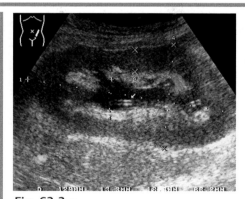

Fig. 63.3 a

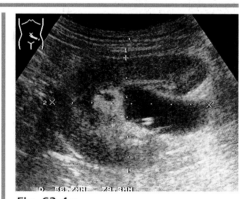

Fig. 63.4 a

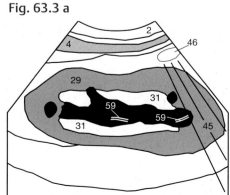

Fig. 63.2 b

Fig. 63.3 b

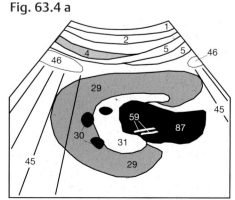

Fig. 63.4 b

These study questions are intended to help you to test your knowledge so you can clear up any comprehension problems or close any gaps before you move on to the next organ system. Pursued with a little determination, you will find the quiz rather enjoyable. You will find the answers on the preceding pages (questions 1 through 5 and 8) or on p. 124 (images 6, 7, and 9).

1. From memory, draw a typical longitudinal section of the right kidney, paying attention to the position of the medullary pyramids relative to the border between the parenchyma and renal pelvis (maximum 2 minutes). Repeat this task for a transverse section of the right kidney at the level of its hilum, and consider its position relative to the liver and the inferior vena cava. Repeat both tasks (important: at intervals of more than 2 hours) until you are able to complete them without any errors.

2. Make a rough sketch showing the different forms of the normal kidney compared with the respective findings in grade I through III urinary obstruction. Discuss the differentiating criteria with a fellow student. Validate your sketches by comparing them with the images on pages 51 and 52.

3. How do you recognize nephrolithiasis? List a few possible underlying disorders that can cause kidney stones. With the help of other sources from the literature, provide a differential diagnosis of hematuria (evidence of blood in the urine).

4. List the sonographic characteristics of a renal angiomyolipoma. What type of tumor is similar to this tumor? Why can it be difficult to differentiate it from other types of tumor?

5. Do you remember the normal values for kidney size, the parenchyma to pelvis (PP) index, and the grades of urinary obstruction in children and adults? Write down your values and compare them with those listed on pages 47, 52, and 55.

6. Carefully examine the ultrasound images in **Figs. 64.1** and **64.2** and write down the imaging planes – all visualized organs, vessels, and muscles – and, of course, your working diagnosis and your reasoning behind it.

Questions with emphasis on pediatrics:

7. **Figure 64.3** is a voiding cystourethrogram (oblique radiograph) of a child's pelvis at the time of voiding. Please examine it closely and state your diagnosis.

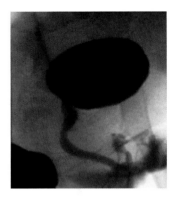

Fig. 64.3

8. How wide can the normal pelvicaliceal system measure in a term newborn? At how many millimeters of pelvic width do you order follow-up examinations or additional imaging studies to exclude a urinary obstruction?

9. This image (**Fig. 64.4**) shows a transverse section of the upper abdomen at the level of the renal vessels. Describe the organs and vessels that you can recognize. Which vessel is atypical in its course and what conclusion do you draw from that?

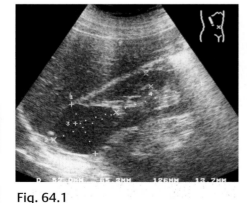

Fig. 64.1

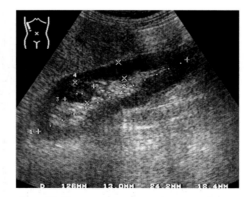

Fig. 64.2

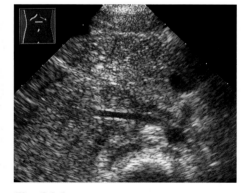

Fig. 64.4

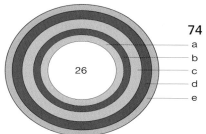
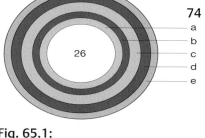

74
a
b
c
d
e

26

Fig. 65.1:
Layers of the stomach wall (74)
a   Mucosa: epithelium
    and lamina propria
b   Mucosa: muscularis mucosae
c   Submucosa
d   Muscular layer (longitudinal
    and circular musculature)
e   Serosa

The normal wall structure of the gastrointestinal (GI) tract consists of five layers, which appear alternatively hyperechoic and hypoechoic (**Fig. 65.1**). The two hypoechoic layers are the muscularis mucosae (**74b**) and the thicker muscular layer or tunica muscularis (**74d**). Under good acoustic conditions or where the stomach (**26**) is filled with water or collapsed, all layers of the wall (**74a-e**) can be identified (**Fig. 65.2**). The anterior aspect of the outer serosal surface (**74e**) appears to merge with the capsule of the liver (**9**), which is also hyperechoic. The posterior serosa cannot always be distinguished from the adjacent pancreas (**33**), depending on the latter's echogenicity.

The width of the gastric wall in adults varies between 5 and 7 mm, depending on its degree of contraction. The hypoechoic muscular layer by itself should not measure more than 5 mm, unless a peristaltic wave passes through it (**Fig. 65.3**). Occasionally, acoustic shadowing (**45**) from gastric air (**47**) can obscure the posterior gastric wall.

In pediatrics, the hypoechoic muscular layer of a term newborn up to 2 months old should not exceed 4 mm. The entire diameter of the pylorus should measure less than 15 mm. Pyloric hypertrophy is present whenever the transverse diameter (**Fig. 65.4**) exceeds these values or the pylorus measures more than 16 mm in length (about 22 mm in the example shown here) in the longitudinal plane (**Fig. 65.5**).

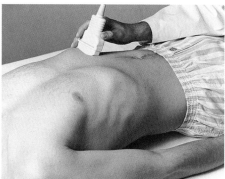
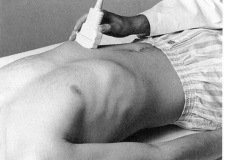
Fig. 65.2 a

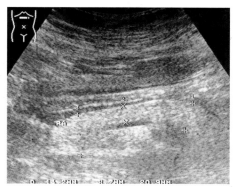
Fig. 65.2 b

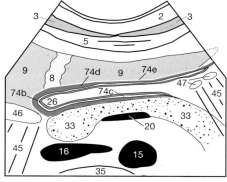
Fig. 65.2 c

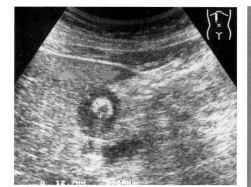
Fig. 65.3 a

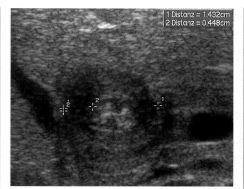
Fig. 65.4 a

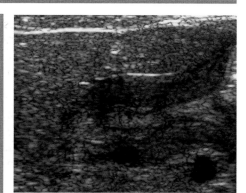
Fig. 65.5 a

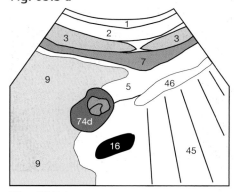
Fig. 65.3 b

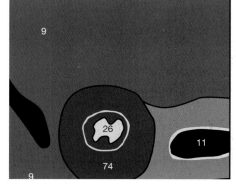
Fig. 65.4 b

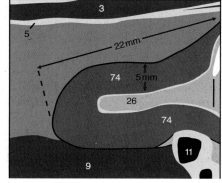
Fig. 65.5 b

P

Gastroesophageal Reflux

To confirm an insufficient lower esophageal sphincter with esophageal reflux in children, the child should be examined after drinking a small amount of fluid or, if it is a newborn, with the stomach filled after nursing. In either case, the fluid invariably contains air bubbles (47) and will be visualized as hyperechoic motion within the stomach (26), often with comet tail artifacts or acoustic shadows (45 in Fig. 66.1). After the esophageal hiatus of the diaphragm is identified in the proper sagittal plane (see Fig. 21.2), one observes the esophagus for some time with head-dependent table positioning to watch for retrograde passage of gastric contents through the cardia and into the esophagus. In adults, it is preferable to perform pulsed fluoroscopy after ingestion of an oral contrast medium.

Gastric Tumors

Malignant focal tumors can invade the normal layers of the stomach wall (see preceding page). A dilated lumen (26) can be an indirect sign of a tumor-induced delay in gastric emptying (Fig. 66.2). In the example shown here, the delayed gastric emptying was caused by a large mural tumor (54) that had invaded the normal layers of the stomach wall and almost completely blocked the lumen.

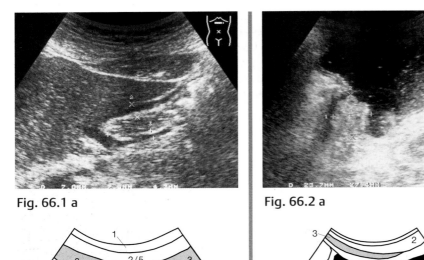

Fig. 66.1 a

Fig. 66.2 a

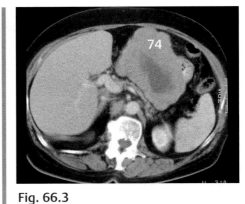

Fig. 66.3

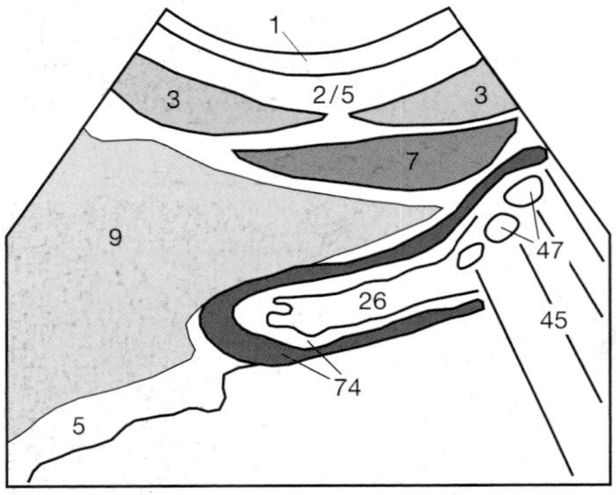

Fig. 66.1 b

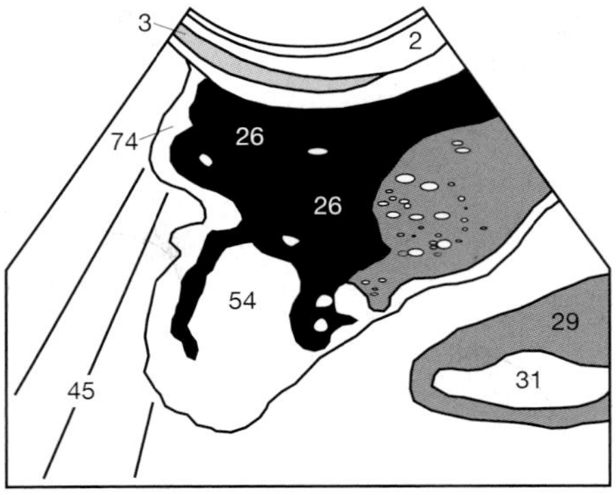

Fig. 66.2 b

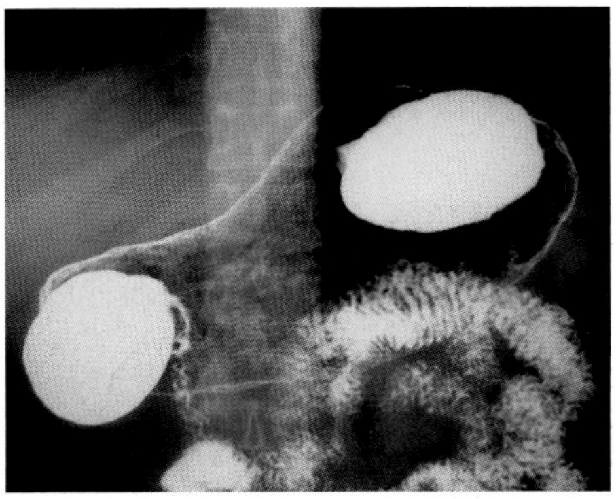

Fig. 66.4

Alternate Imaging Modalities

Since gastric air often prevents complete visualization of the stomach on ultrasound images, other diagnostic modalities are often applied.

Computed Tomography (CT)

The advantage of CT is its superiority in identifying any thickening of the layers of the stomach wall (74), as in the diffuse lymphomatous infiltration of the stomach shown in Fig. 66.3. CT also allows precise evaluation of infiltration of regional lymph nodes and other adjacent organs, regardless of the amount of air in the gastrointestinal tract. However, invasive gastroscopy is still needed to determine the histology of the tumor.

Upper GI Series

A double contrast upper GI series is obtained early in the morning before gastric secretions into the empty stomach interfere with achieving a good coating of contrast medium (e.g., barium sulfate or water-soluble Gastrografin®). The patient first drinks the contrast agent, turns over in a full circle on the examining table, and takes an effervescent powder that releases CO_2 when it comes into contact with water. The CO_2 distends the stomach and allows the examiner to search the mucosal folds under fluoroscopy for lesions, rigid segments, and ulcer craters (Fig. 66.4). Can you tell how this patient with normal findings was positioned? Left or right lateral decubitus, supine, or head-down position? The distribution of contrast medium in the stomach indicates the patient's position. The answer is found on page 125.

Small bowel loops are often very poorly visualized because their walls are normally so thin that they are obscured by the acoustic shadow of intestinal gas. In inflammatory bowel disease, however, the wall becomes thickened at the expense of the intestinal lumen and as a result is better visualized. Ultrasound allows the examiner to observe the dynamics of intestinal peristalsis in real time. With a little patience, one can readily identify atonic segments (lacking peristalsis) or prestenotic hyperperistalsis.

Crohn Disease

This disease frequently affects the terminal ileum (terminal ileitis). The affected bowel segment shows edematous wall thickening (74) and is easily distinguishable from adjacent uninvolved loops (46 in **Fig. 67.1**). Advanced disease can cause such a massively thickened bowel wall (**Fig. 67.2**) that on transverse images it can easily be misinterpreted as a tumorous mass or intussusception (see p. 68). The term "target sign" is commonly used to describe the appearance of the concentric rings of the thickened edematous wall. One should always examine adjacent spaces and the pouch of Douglas (**Fig. 60.4**) for free intra-abdominal fluid that can be a sign of perforation. Long segments of mural thickening can be due to causes other than inflammation, such as diffuse lymphomatous infiltration of the bowel, which is frequently encountered in immunosuppressed patients.

The connections of individual small bowel loops to the root of the mesentery are normally not identifiable but can be delineated in the presence of extensive lymphadenopathy or massive ascites (**Fig. 67.3**). The oblique section of the small bowel loop (46) shown here appears to float in ascites (68), which is devoid of internal echoes (possibly due to hemorrhage) except for reverberation artifacts (51a) from the anterior abdominal wall (2, 3).

Hernias

Protrusion of a bowel loop (46) through the anterior abdominal fascia (6) can be observed around the umbilicus (**Fig. 67.4**) and along the linea alba. The width of the hernia (⟷) is a crucial determinant of the risk of incarceration. A wide hernia is less likely to impinge on the vessels supplying the herniated bowel loop (120). One should be alert to ischemic thickening of the wall of the herniated bowel loop (74) as it is an important indirect sign of hypoperfusion (not present in the example shown).

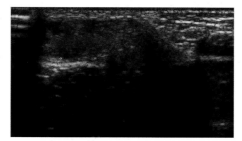

Fig. 67.4 a

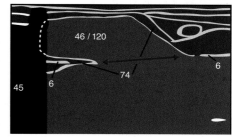

Fig. 67.4 b

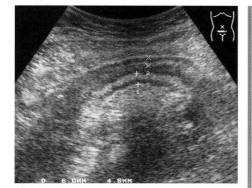

Fig. 67.1 a

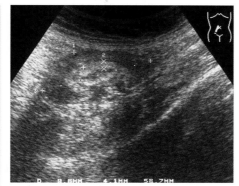

Fig. 67.2 a

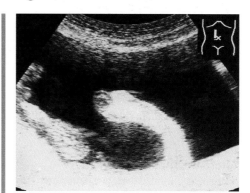

Fig. 67.3 a

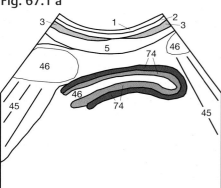

Fig. 67.1 b

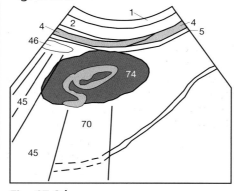

Fig. 67.2 b

Fig. 67.3 b

Intussusception

Intussusception in the newborn is most likely to occur at the age of 6 to 9 months. Males are more frequently affected than females. The rule of thumb is that intussusception very rarely occurs before the age of 3 months and after the age of 3 years. The patient typically experiences episodic pain of abrupt onset with little or no pain between episodes. Usually, the terminal ileum prolapses through the ileocecal valve into the colon, so that a circular bowel wall lies within lumen of the colon (**Figs. 68.1** and **68.2**). Intussusception involving the jejunum is less common.

The intussusception produces an external hypoechoic muscular layer (**74d**) separated from the prolapsed inner muscular layer by the hyperechoic mucosa (**74b**). Its cross section shows concentric rings, referred to as "target" or "bull's eye sign." Occasionally, the two echogenic mucosal layers (**74b**) of both bowel segments are visualized (**Fig. 68.2**). **Fig. 68.3** shows how an intussusception (**74**) appears on a CT scan, visualized here next to fluid-filled colonic segments (**43**).

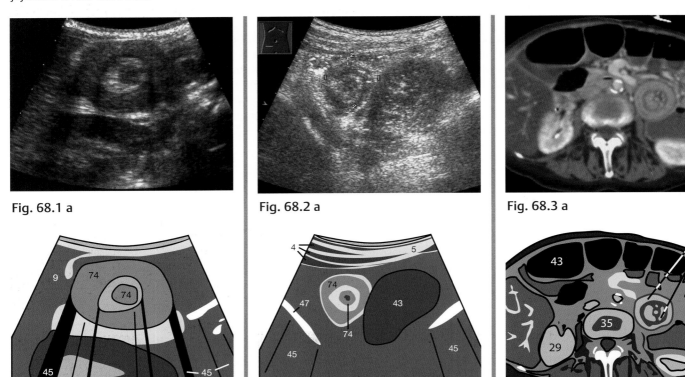

Fig. 68.1 a

Fig. 68.2 a

Fig. 68.3 a

Fig. 68.1 b

Fig. 68.2 b

Fig. 68.3 b

Contrast Enema

Whenever an intussusception has been confirmed by either method, reduction of the intussuscepted bowel segment (➘) should be immediately attempted by means of a contrast enema (**Fig. 68.4**). This is necessary in order to promptly prevent or resolve compression of the vessels of the involved mesenteric root. In the example shown, the small bowel was already intussuscepted as far as the mid transverse colon.

Ideally, the hydrostatic pressure of the retrograde injection of contrast medium completely pushes back the intussuscepted intestinal segment, so the child is spared a surgical intervention. The ultrasound follow-up examination after reduction is important. There should be no evidence of a target sign. Occasionally, intussusception recurs after successful reduction and must be treated by a repeat contrast enema or by surgery.

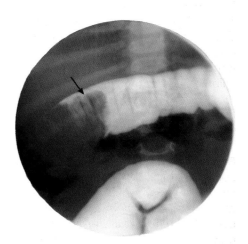

Fig. 68.4

Appendicitis

A normal vermiform appendix has an inner hyperechoic layer surrounded by an outer hypoechoic layer (**Fig. 69.1**). The maximum diameter of a normal appendix should not measure more than 6 mm and the wall should be no more than 2 mm thick. Measurements of 7 mm and 3 mm or more, respectively, are pathologic.

Additionally, acute appendicitis typically causes edematous wall thickening, which appears as a hypoechoic ring with a hyperechoic center (mucosa and narrowed lumen) in the transverse plane (**Fig. 69.2a**). In the longitudinal plane (**Fig. 69.2b**), the thickened appendix can be distinguished from other bowel segments by its lack of peristalsis and its dead end. One can also test for local tenderness by gently applying pressure with the transducer. The perifocal bowel loops can show a reactive reduction in peristalsis. An abscess presents as an increasingly inhomogeneous and hyperechoic conglomeration that in its late stage makes the appendix difficult to identify.

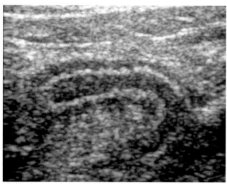

Fig. 69.1

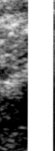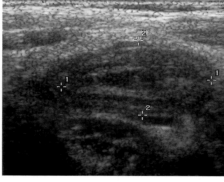

Fig. 69.2 a

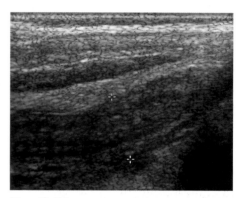

Fig. 69.2 b

Appendix, Normal Values		
	Normal	**Inflammatory**
Wall thickness	≤ 2 mm	≥ 3 mm
Maximum external diameter	≤ 6 mm	≥ 7 mm

Diarrhea

In watery diarrhea, the bowel loops contain a large amount of anechoic fluid (**46** in **Fig. 69.3**). These intraluminal fluid accumulations should not be mistaken for extraluminal ascites (see **Fig. 67.3**). In fecal impaction (**Fig. 70.1**) or Hirschsprung disease, the bowel contents are more echogenic.

Hirschsprung Disease

The toxic megacolon of Hirschsprung disease is characterized by an aganglionic colonic segment with a narrowed lumen and massive dilation of the colonic segment proximal to it (**43**), whose luminal width differs significantly from adjacent bowel loops (**46** in **Fig. 69.4**).

Familial clustering involves boys in about 80% of all cases. A typical funnel-shaped junction is observed between the narrowed segment and the megacolon. Often the dilated lumen contains only a little intestinal gas (**47**) with distal acoustic shadowing (**45**), allowing good sound transmission through the retained fecal matter.

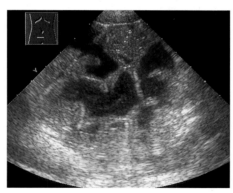

Fig. 69.3 a

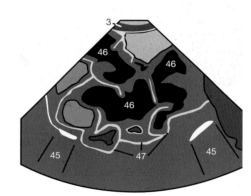

Fig. 69.3 b

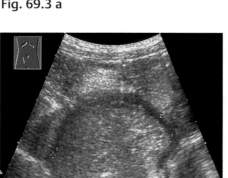

Fig. 69.4 a

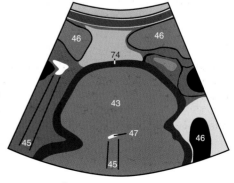

Fig. 69.4 b

P

Fecal Impaction

Normally, only the wall of the colon near the transducer can be evaluated because the colon contains so much gas that the lumen or opposite wall cannot be evaluated. However, fecal material is occasionally retained, especially in older patients (fecal impaction, **Fig. 70.1**). Here it is seen in the transverse colon (43) without gas, allowing good evaluation of both walls of the colon.

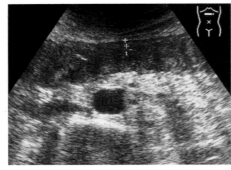

Fig. 70.1 a

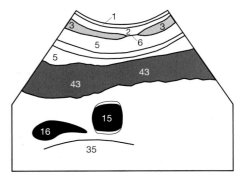

Fig. 70.1 b

Colitis

In inflammatory thickening of the colonic wall (74) in the setting of colitis, the edematous semilunar folds can become much more prominent than usual, as seen here in the sigmoid colon (**Fig. 70.2**). Alternatively, thickening of the colonic wall can be ischemic, as is seen in mesenteric infarction or mesenteric venous thrombosis.

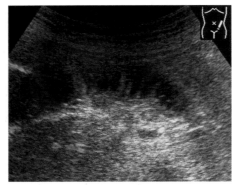

Fig. 70.2 a

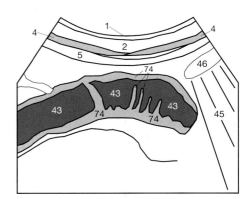

Fig. 70.2 b

Diverticulitis

One possible complication of a colonic diverticulum is circumscribed diverticulitis. **Fig. 70.3** shows the neck of the diverticulum (*) between the normal lumen (43) and the hypoechoic diverticulum (54). Note the thickened colonic wall (74) which is also seen on the CT of the same patient (**Fig. 70.4**). The rectosigmoid junction (43) in the center is still clearly distinguishable from the adjacent fatty tissue whereas the fatty tissue immediately adjacent to the diverticulum (54) is not clearly demarcated and shows edematous thickening (white arrows). **Fig. 70.5** shows gas (47) in a small diverticulum with thickening of the adjacent bowel wall (74) in early stage diverticulitis.

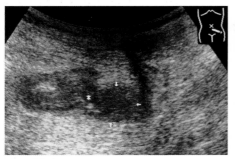

Fig. 70.3 a

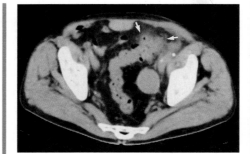

Fig. 70.4 a

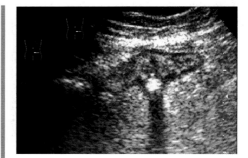

Fig. 70.5 a

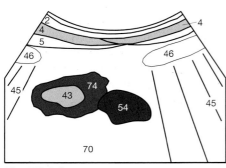

Fig. 70.3 b

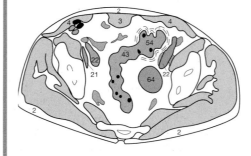

Fig. 70.4 b

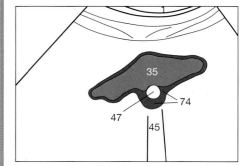

Fig. 70.5 b

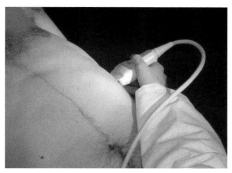

Fig. 71.1

Examination Technique

The spleen is primarily visualized with the patient supine. It is best to have the patient lie close to the left edge of the examining table. This makes it easier to apply the transducer parallel to the widened intercostal space from a posterolateral position **(Fig. 71.1)**. The examiner should stand up or sit on the right edge of the examining table to have adequate reach. The examination is performed in expiration to exclude the left lung base **(47)** and eliminate any acoustic shadowing **(45)** that may obscure the spleen **(37 in Fig. 71.2)**. Often the part of the spleen just beneath the diaphragm **(13)** is poorly visualized. Alternatively, one can perform the examination with the patient in the right lateral decubitus position **(Fig. 71.2a)**, but the supine position is usually better. The lower pole of the spleen may occasionally be obscured by acoustic shadows of adjacent bowel loops **(43)**.

Spleen Size

The normal adult spleen measures about 4 cm x 7 cm x 11 cm (the "4711 rule"), whereby the longitudinal dimension **(L)** can be as much as 13 cm (instead of 11 cm) without any clinical significance, for instance, in patients who have had infectious mononucleosis. The thickness or diameter **(D**, measured from the hilum to the diaphragmatic capsule of the spleen) provides more information: If it exceeds 6 cm (instead of 4 cm), additional tests are indicated to exclude a lymphatic disorder, unless venous congestion is present due to portal hypertension.

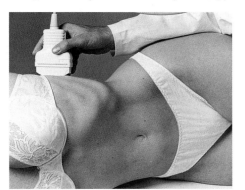

Fig. 71.2 a

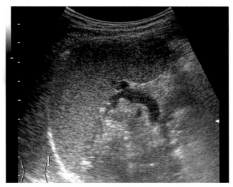

Fig. 71.2 b

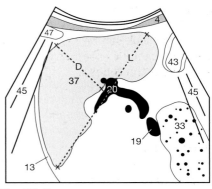

Fig. 71.2 c

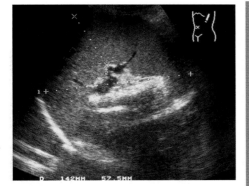

Fig. 71.3 a

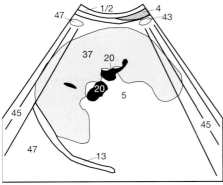

Fig. 71.3 b

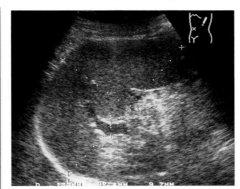

Fig. 71.4 a

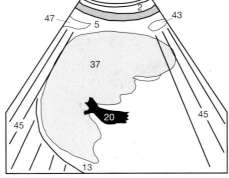

Fig. 71.4 b

Curtain Trick

In some patients, the cranial spleen **(37)** is obscured by acoustic shadows **(45)**, either spontaneously or after deep inspiration where the lung **(47)** extends too far into the costodiaphragmatic recess **(Fig. 71.3)**. In this situation, one can take advantage of the fact that the spleen will return to its cranial position more slowly than the lung during measured but swift expiration following maximum inspiration. This relative motion makes the acoustic shadow recede like a "curtain." The examiner has to wait for the right moment and then tell the patient to immediately hold his or her breath. This maneuver often succeeds in visualizing the regions of the spleen immediately beneath the diaphragm (along the left edge of the image in **Fig. 71.4**).

Many disorders are accompanied by diffuse, homogeneous enlargement of the spleen. The differential diagnosis includes portal hypertension (Fig. 72.2), in which the splenic vein (20) is dilated and its branches prominent at the splenic hilum. Acute viral infection or even a previous infection with Epstein–Barr virus can produce splenomegaly. In some cases, infectious mononucleosis can resolve and leave behind slight–to–moderate splenomegaly for life without any clinical significance.

Systemic Hematologic Disorders

Splenomegaly typically accompanies systemic hematologic diseases, such as acute or chronic lymphatic leukemia (CLL). Fig. 72.1 was obtained in a leukemia patient and shows a spleen with an adjacent accessory spleen (86) and the tail of the pancreas (33) close to the splenic hilum. In principle, any disorder involving increased turnover of erythrocytes, such as a hemolytic anemia or polycythemia vera, can cause splenomegaly. In such cases the spleen may be grossly enlarged, even extending into the pelvis (Fig. 72.3), and may exhibit focal infarcts (see Fig. 73.1). The "kissing phenomenon" may also be observed, in which the massively enlarged spleen displaces the stomach and extends as far as the left lobe of the liver.

When evaluating the spleen, it is important to be alert to any signs of thickening. The original crescentic or half moon shape with tapered poles is lost, and the poles appear rounded or thickened (Fig. 72.1). Ectopic splenic tissue in the bed of the spleen, occasionally present as a remnant of embryonic development, can also become hypertrophic when stimulated.

Consequently, visible accessory spleens (86) at the hilum (Fig. 72.1) or lower splenic pole are not uncommon in diffuse splenomegaly. They have the same echogenicity as the remaining splenic parenchyma (37) and are sharply demarcated. However, they can be difficult to differentiate from enlarged lymph nodes (55) as illustrated in Fig. 72.3.

Practical Suggestion

Neither size nor echogenicity of the enlarged spleen reveals the nature of the underlying disease. If the ultrasound examination of the abdomen unexpectedly detects splenomegaly, all accessible nodal groups (para-aortic, portal, iliac, and cervical nodes) should be examined for lymphadenopathy suggestive of a systemic hematologic disorder. Portal hypertension should also be excluded by measuring the diameter of the splenic vein (normal value < 10 mm), portal vein (normal value < 15 mm), and superior mesenteric vein, and by searching for portocaval collaterals at the porta hepatis.

Spleen size should be documented as accurately as possible to allow follow-up examinations to determine whether size has increased or decreased, such as can occur after resolution of a viral infection or secondary to chemotherapy in the interim, depending on the underlying disease. Keep this in mind when you perform the initial examination.

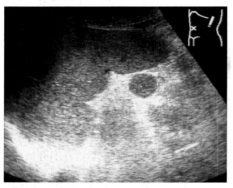

Fig. 72.1 a

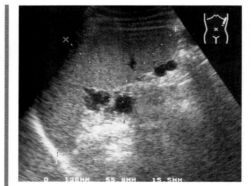

Fig. 72.2 a

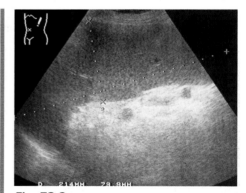

Fig. 72.3 a

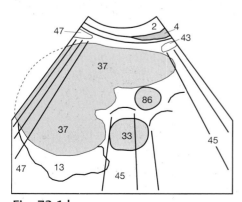

Fig. 72.1 b

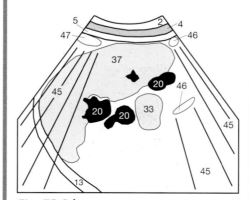

Fig. 72.2 b

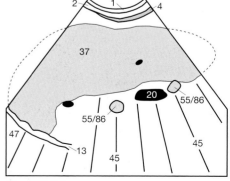

Fig. 72.3 b

Splenic Infarcts

Focal infarcts **(71)** are especially likely to occur in the setting of rapidly progressive splenomegaly. Early-stage infarcts appear as hypoechoic areas within perfused hyperechoic areas **(Fig. 73.1)**. Supplemental color duplex sonography can establish the status of splenic perfusion quickly and noninvasively.

Lymphomatous Infiltration

Non-Hodgkin lymphoma can present with an isolated hypoechoic splenic lesion or there may be inhomogeneous involvement of the entire spleen. An enlarged spleen that appears homogeneous on conventional ultrasound scans can nevertheless contain lymphomatous focal lesions that escape detection. The detection rate has increased markedly with the introduction of echo-enhancing contrast media used in combination with harmonic imaging (see p. 12).

Splenic Hematomas

Definitive exclusion of splenic hematomas is of utmost importance in trauma patients as an acute hemorrhage may initially be contained within the splenic capsule (intracapsular or subcapsular injury). The splenic capsule may rupture only after some delay (in about 50% of all cases within the first week), precipitating a life-threatening hemorrhage into the abdominal cavity (delayed splenic rupture). Therefore, one must carefully examine any hypoechoic lesion or delicate hypoechoic double contour of the splenic capsule to exclude such an injury. Some splenic hematomas **(50)** are also inhomogeneous **(Fig. 73.2)** or isoechoic to the surrounding splenic parenchyma **(37)**. The arrow (◄) in **Fig. 73.2** indicates the site where you should search for anechoic intra-abdominal fluid (indicative of hemorrhage) in the supine patient. The site is along the abdominal aspect of the diaphragm **(13)**, posterior to the upper pole of the spleen.

Hyperechoic Lesions

Spherical and homogeneous hyperechoic lesions that are sharply demarcated from the splenic parenchyma generally represent benign splenic hemangiomas, with features identical to those of hepatic hemangiomas **(Fig. 39.2)**. Such findings may also represent hyperechoic calcifications secondary to tuberculosis infection or cirrhosis of the liver. Multiple hyperechoic focal lesions **(53)** give the spleen the appearance of a "starry sky" **(Fig. 73.3)**. Such lesions also occur as postinfectious scarring. Splenic abscesses and the rare splenic metastases can exhibit a rather varied ultrasound morphology, depending on age and immune status. Unfortunately there are no simple, reliable ultrasound criteria for differential diagnosis.

Splenic Cysts

Congenital splenic cysts are anechoic and less common than hepatic cysts. Their appearance on ultrasound does not differ from hepatic cysts (see p. 39). Acquired splenic cysts develop secondary to trauma or infarction, or in the setting of parasitic infestation. **Fig.73.4** shows a CT with cysts containing obvious radial septa (◥) in the setting of echinococcosis of the liver and spleen.

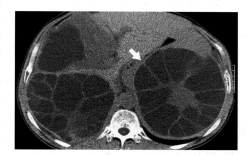

Fig. 73.4

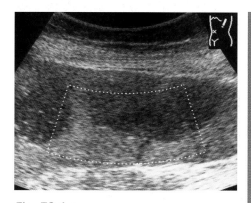

Fig. 73.1 a

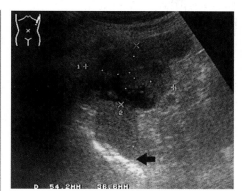

Fig. 73.2 a

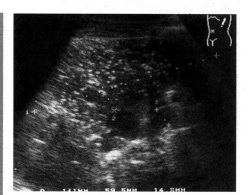

Fig. 73.3 a

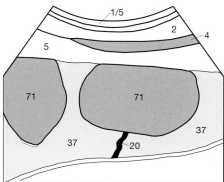

Fig. 73.1 b

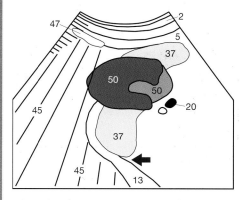

Fig. 73.2 b

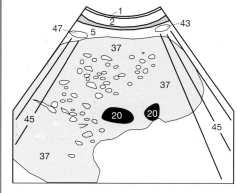

Fig. 73.3 b

Splenic Size in Pediatrics

While the "4711 rule" applies to adults with the caveats discussed above, the size of the spleen in children is measured craniocaudally along the mid-axillary line (not parallel to the inter-costal space), and is specified relative to height (according to Weitzel, D.: Sonographic Organometrics in Childhood, Mainz).

Height [cm]	Length of spleen [cm]		
	$\overline{m} - 2\,SD$	$\overline{m}$	$\overline{m} + 2\,SD$
Newborn	2.90	4.07	5.24
< 55	2.13	2.91	3.69
55 – 70	2.44	3.46	4.48
71 – 85	2.23	3.71	5.19
86 – 100	2.61	4.69	6.77
101 – 110	3.02	4.88	6.74
111 – 120	3.38	5.26	7.14
121 – 130	3.37	5.31	7.25
131 – 140	4.10	5.96	7.82
141 – 150	4.61	5.81	7.01
> 150	4.36	6.18	8.00

Spleen: Quiz for Self Evaluation

In our ultrasound courses for students and physicians, the sonographic evaluation of the spleen is invariably found to be particularly challenging. It is interesting to note that more than 90% of all participants initially place the transducer along the anterior (not posterior) axillary line and run into difficulties with acoustic shadowing of the colon or small bowel. Therefore, practice the correct visualization with your partner and keep in mind the necessity of standing up to extend your reach.

Here are the other learning points (you will find the answers to quiz questions 1 to 4 on the preceding pages and the answer to the image quiz at the end of the book on page 124):

1. Write down the normal size measurements of the spleen in adults, and put the significance of splenomegaly in perspective.

2. What trick do you know to visualize the subdiaphragmatic aspect of the spleen when you encounter superimposed pulmonary air? How does it work?

3. Imagine you have a patient with multiple injuries who has or may have sustained blunt abdominal trauma. What do you look for on ultrasound, and where do you place the transducer for that purpose?

4. You unexpectedly discover splenomegaly. How do you proceed?

5. Systematically evaluate the following image. Proceed in the order recommended in the primer on ultrasound on page 116 to give your thoughts proper direction.

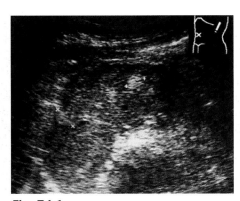

Fig. 74.1

Prostate Gland

Transabdominal sonography of the reproductive organs requires a full bladder (38) to displace gas-filled bowel loops (46) superiorly and laterally and prevent their acoustic shadows (45) from interfering with visualization. The prostate gland (42) is at the bladder floor anterior to the rectum (43) and is visualized in suprapubic transverse and sagittal planes (Fig. 75.1).

Prostatic Hypertrophy

The normal prostate gland should not measure more than 5 cm x 3 cm x 3 cm and its calculated volume should not exceed 25 mL (A x B x C x 0.5). A high percentage of older men have prostatic hypertrophy (Fig. 75.2), which can cause voiding difficulties and trabeculation of the bladder (Fig. 60.2). An enlarged prostate gland (42) elevates and indents the floor of the bladder (38). The bladder wall (77) is usually well demarcated and appears as a smooth, hyperechoic line (Fig. 75.2).

Prostate cancer (54) generally arises in the periphery of the gland. It can invade the bladder wall and eventually protrude into the bladder lumen (Fig. 75.3). Increasing urethral compression can lead to hypertrophy of the musculature of the bladder wall (77), which then appears thickened (Fig. 75.3).

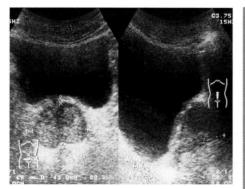

Fig. 75.1 a

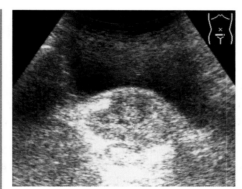

Fig. 75.2 a

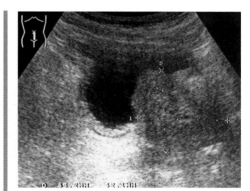

Fig. 75.3 a

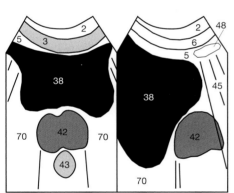

Fig. 75.1 b

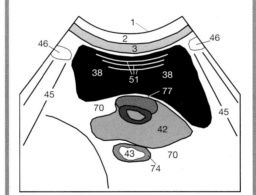

Fig. 75.2 b

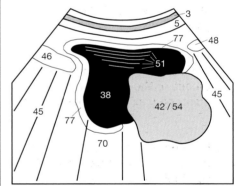

Fig. 75.3 b

Testes and Scrotum

The adult testis (98) is normally homogeneously hypoechoic and clearly demarcated from the layers of the scrotum (100). It measures about 3 cm x 4 cm in the longitudinal plane (Fig. 75.4). The upper pole of the testis is covered by the epididymis (99), which extends along the surface of the testis. In children, an undescended testis should be excluded on the transverse image (see p. 76), which must show both testes next to each other in the scrotum.

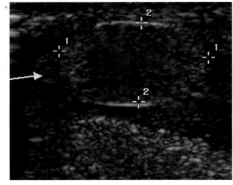

Fig. 75.4 a

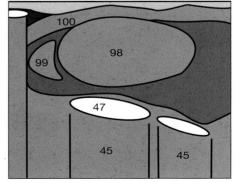

Fig. 75.4 b

Undescended Testis

If both testes are not found in the scrotum at 3 months, the undescended or ectopic testis must be located. The testis **(98)** is frequently found in the inguinal canal near the abdominal wall **(2/5)** as shown in **Fig. 76.1**. If the testis cannot be located on ultrasound, a supplementary MRI scan is indicated as malignant degeneration can occur in an undescended or ectopic testis.

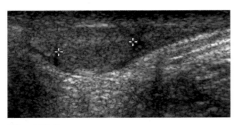

Fig. 76.1 a

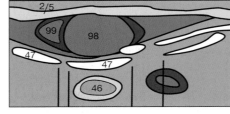

Fig. 76.1 b

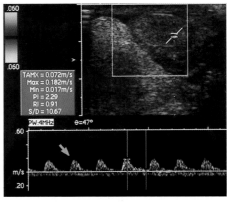

Fig. 76.2

Orchitis and Epididymitis

The differential diagnosis of sudden-onset severe scrotal pain that radiates into the inguinal region must consider testicular torsion in addition to testicular or epididymal infection. Testicular tissue can tolerate ischemia for only about 6 hours before irreversible necrosis sets in. In an infection, Doppler sonography shows perfusion with arterial pulses in the flow profile (↘ in **Fig. 76.2**), and the affected side may even show hyperperfusion. Torsion leads to considerably reduced or absent testicular perfusion in comparison with the contralateral testis.

Orchitis or epididymitis typically shows edematous enlargement of the testis **(98)** or epididymis **(99)** as well as thickening of multiple layers of the scrotal wall **(100)**, as shown in **Fig. 76.3**. Equivocal findings can be resolved by contralateral comparison.

Hydrocele and Inguinal Hernia

A homogeneous anechoic fluid accumulation **(Fig. 76.4)** is either a hydrocele **(64)** or a varicocele. A varicocele enlarges with the Valsalva maneuver and shows flow on color duplex sonography. Occasionally, a herniated bowel loop **(46)** is seen in the inguinal canal or scrotum together with a hydrocele **(64)** next to the normal testis **(98, Fig. 76.5)**.

Malignant testicular tumors usually produce inhomogeneous changes in the testicular parenchyma. Malignant but still well-differentiated seminomas can be homogeneous with mostly unremarkable ultrasound morphology.

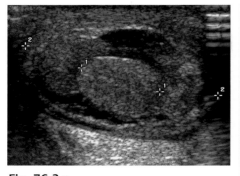

Fig. 76.3 a

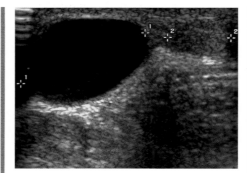

Fig. 76.4 a

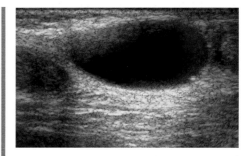

Fig. 76.5 a

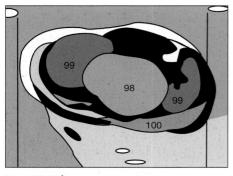

Fig. 76.3 b

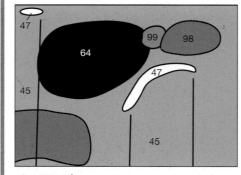

Fig. 76.4 b

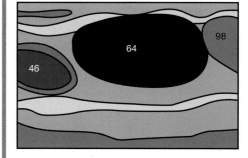

Fig. 76.5 b

The transabdominal visualization (Fig. 77.1) of the uterus (39) including ovaries (91), vagina (41), and rectum (43) requires a full bladder as an acoustic window. Because of the depth of penetration required, lower frequencies around 3.5 MHz are used with correspondingly limited resolution. Gynecologists often prefer intracavitary ultrasound as an alternative because of the higher spatial resolution (see below).

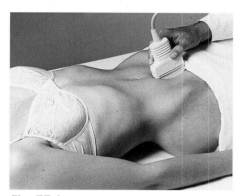

Fig. 77.1 a

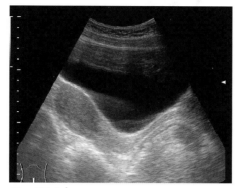

Fig. 77.1 b

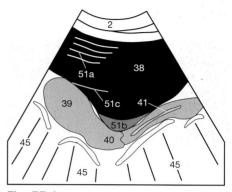

Fig. 77.1 c

Endovaginal Ultrasound

Because of the proximity to the target organs, transvaginal transducers (Fig. 77.2) can be operated at a higher frequency (5–10 MHz or more) with correspondingly higher spatial resolution (see p. 9). Another advantage of endovaginal ultrasound is that the bladder need not be full. An assortment of electronic and mechanical transducers with variable imaging sectors (70–180°) is available. Transducers that emit an eccentric sound beam must be rotated 180° to visualize the contralateral ovary.

In contrast to transabdominal imaging, the caudocranial endovaginal scan images findings "upside down." The sound waves propagate from the bottom to the top of the image (Fig. 77.3). This orientation visualizes intestinal loops with acoustic shadows (45) in the upper half of the image, whereas the uterus (39) and cervical region (40) are visualized in the lower half near the transducer.

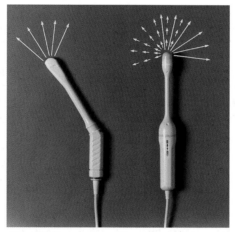

Fig. 77.2 a

Image Orientation

Most gynecologists prefer sagittal planes viewed from the patient's left side, the opposite of the convention used by internists. The bladder (38) and other anterior anatomic structures are on the left side of the image (Fig. 77.3) whereas the cervix (40) and other posterior structures are on the right side.

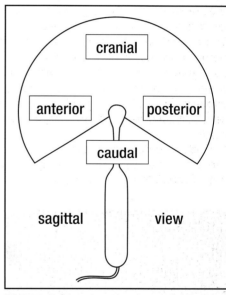

Fig. 77.2 b

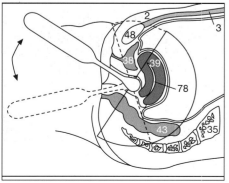

Fig. 77.3 a

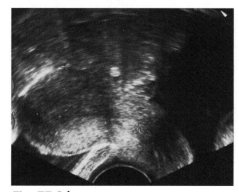

Fig. 77.3 b

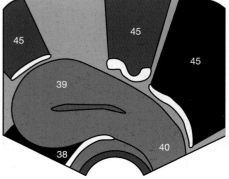

Fig. 77.3 c

Uterus: Normal Findings

The thickness of the endometrium (78) varies with the menstrual cycle. Immediately after menstruation, only a thin hyperechoic central line is observed (**Fig. 78.1**). Around the time of ovulation, the endometrium (78) is demarcated from the myometrium (39) by a thin hyperechoic rim (☛ in **Fig. 78.2**). After ovulation, the secretory endometrium increasingly loses its central echo (➡ in **Fig. 78.3**) until the endometrium becomes entirely hyperechoic.

The normally homogeneous hyperechoic myometrium can be

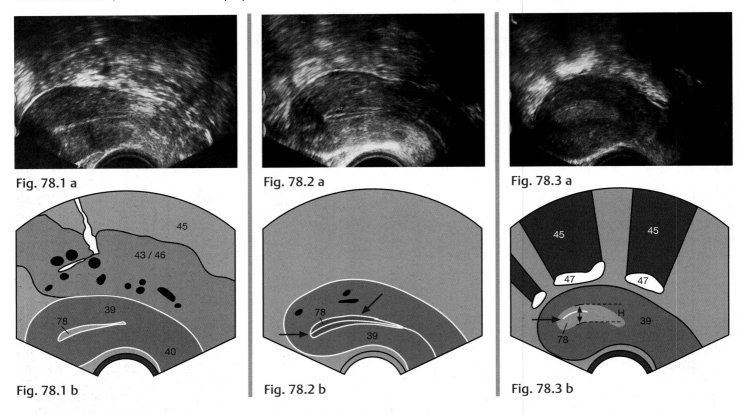

Fig. 78.1 a

Fig. 78.2 a

Fig. 78.3 a

Fig. 78.1 b

Fig. 78.2 b

Fig. 78.3 b

traversed by vessels appearing as anechoic areas. The body (39) and cervix (40) of the uterus do not differ in echogenicity. In premenopausal women, 2 times the height (**H**) of the endometrium (78) should be less than 15 mm (**Fig. 78.3**). In postmenopausal women, that measurement should be less than 6 mm, unless the patient is undergoing hormone replacement therapy. To avoid exaggerating size due to oblique sectioning, the measurements should be obtained exclusively on longitudinal sections of the uterus.

Intrauterine Device (IUD)

An IUD (92) is easily recognized by its high echogenicity with acoustic shadowing (45) and should be located at the fundus in the uterine cavity. The distance between the IUD (d) and the fundal extension of the endometrium should be less than 5 mm, and the distance to the end of the fundus (D) less than 20 mm (**Fig. 78.4**). Longer distances (**Fig. 78.5**) suggest the IUD is displaced toward the cervix (40) and is no longer providing sufficient contraceptive protection.

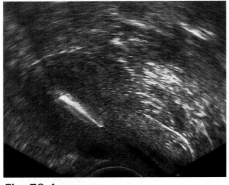

Fig. 78.4 a

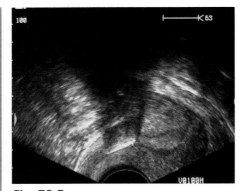

Fig. 78.5 a

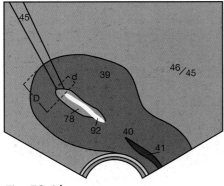

Fig. 78.4 b

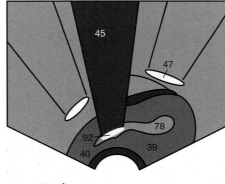

Fig. 78.5 b

The normal uterus is demarcated by hyperechoic serosa and shows a homogeneous hypoechoic myometrium (39). Myomas (54) are the most common benign uterine tumors. They arise from the smooth musculature and usually occur in the uterine body. For preoperative planning of a myomectomy, myomas are categorized as intramural / transmural (Fig. 79.1), submucosal (Fig. 79.2), or subserosal projecting from the outer uterine surface (Fig. 79.3). A submucosal myoma can easily be mistaken for endometrial polyps (65 in Fig. 79.2).

Myomas exhibit a homogeneous or concentric crescentic echo pattern and are sharply demarcated with a smooth surface. However, they can also contain calcifications with acoustic shadowing or central necroses. The size of myomas should be accurately measured and documented on follow-up to exclude rapid progression indicative of rare sarcomatous degeneration. Note that sudden enlargement of a myoma in early pregnancy can be benign in nature.

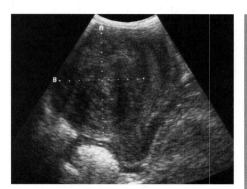

Fig. 79.1 a

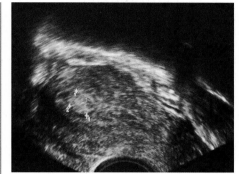

Fig. 79.2 a

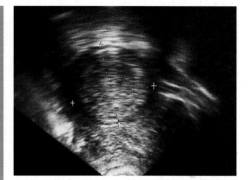

Fig. 79.3 a

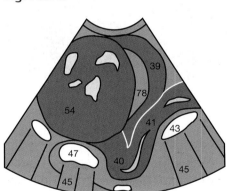

Fig. 79.1 b

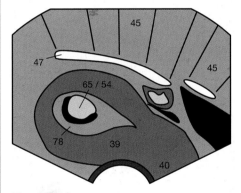

Fig. 79.2 b

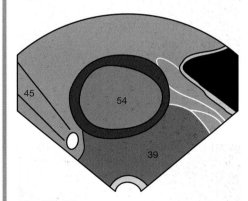

Fig. 79.3 b

Postmenopausal endometrial hyperplasia (Fig. 79.4) can be induced by administration of estrogens, by estrogen-secreting ovarian tumors, or persistent follicles. Persistently high estrogen levels increase the risk of the endometrial hyperplasia degenerating into an adenocarcinoma (54 in Fig. 79.6). Malignant criteria include an endometrium that measures more than 6 mm

after and 15 mm before menopause, exhibits an inhomogeneous echo pattern, and is irregularly demarcated as in Fig. 79.6.
A hypoechoic accumulation of blood (✒) in the uterine cavity (hematometra) can be caused by postinflammatory adhesions in the cervical canal following conization or by a cervical tumor (Fig. 79.5).

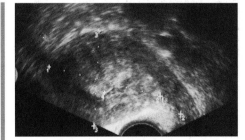

Fig. 79.6 a

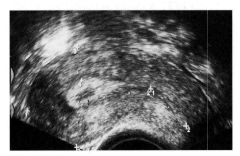

Fig. 79.4

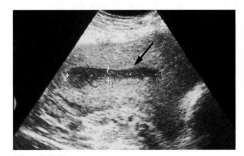

Fig. 79.5

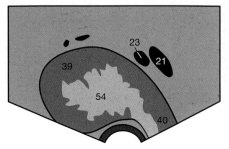

Fig. 79.6 b

Volume Measurement

The ovaries (91) are visualized in a craniolateral sagittal plane (Fig. 80.1) and are usually located in the immediate vicinity of the iliac vessels (21 and 22). To measure volume, the ovaries are also visualized in a transverse plane. The product of the three diameters multiplied by 0.5 provides an adequate estimate of ovarian volume. In adults, the values range from 5.5 to 10 cm³, with a mean of 8 cm³. Ovarian volume is not affected by pregnancies, but continuously decreases in postmenopausal women from about 3.5 to 2.5 cm³, depending on the length of time since menopause.

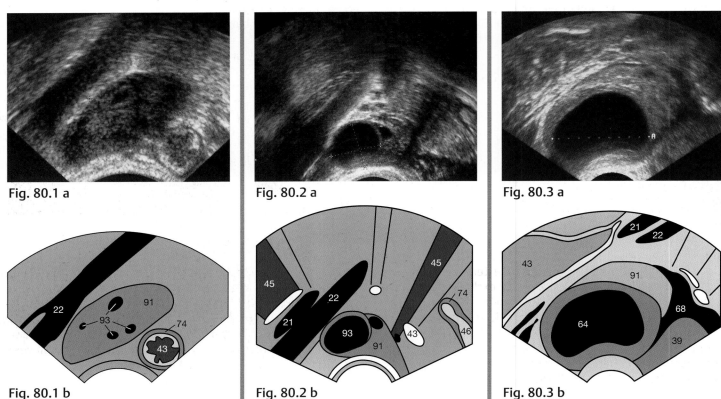

Fig. 80.1 a   Fig. 80.2 a   Fig. 80.3 a

Fig. 80.1 b   Fig. 80.2 b   Fig. 80.3 b

Cycle Phases

In the first days of a new cycle, several follicles (93) are normally visible as small 4–6 mm anechoic cysts within the ovary. Beginning with the 10th day of the cycle (Fig. 80.2), a dominant follicle (Graafian follicle) measuring about 10 mm in diameter begins to mature. It shows linear growth of about 2 mm per day, reaching a preovulatory diameter of 1.8 cm to 2.5 cm. This process is accompanied by regression of the remaining follicles.

For infertility treatment and in vitro fertilization (IVF), ultrasound follow-up examinations performed at close intervals can trace follicular maturation and occasionally even demonstrate the time of ovulation. Follicle size exceeding 2 cm, demonstration of a small mural ovarian cumulus, and digitations within the follicular wall are regarded as signs of imminent ovulation. Following the ovulation, the Graafian follicle disappears or at least markedly decreases in size. At the same time, free fluid may be detectable in the pouch of Douglas.

Vascular proliferation into the ruptured follicle transforms it into the progesterone-producing yellow body (corpus luteum), which remains visible for only a few days as a hyperechoic area at the site of the former follicle. If nidation occurs, the corpus luteum persists and can remain visible as a corpus luteum cyst (64) up to the 14th week of pregnancy (Fig. 80.3).

Abnormalities of follicular development include premature follicular luteinization leading to missed ovulation and formation of a follicular cyst (64 in Fig. 80.4). Remember that a follicular cyst that remains larger than 3 mm for more than one menstrual cycle may represent a persistent follicle (see next page).

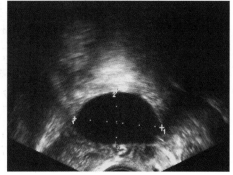

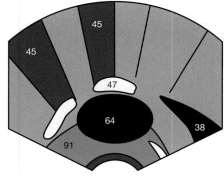

Fig. 80.4 a   Fig. 80.4 b

An ovarian cyst exceeding 5 cm in diameter (see p. 80) is suspicious for tumor. Malignancy must be suspected especially where a cyst exhibits septa and/or solid internal echoes (↖) or increased wall thickness **(Fig. 81.1)**. Similar features are found in dermoid cysts **(Fig. 81.2)**, which account for 15% of unilateral ovarian tumors. Their internal echoes (↘) correspond to sebum, hair, and other tissue components. They are

usually benign and only rarely become malignant.

These findings must be distinguished from hemorrhagic or endometriotic cysts, which either contain fluid levels (→) within their lumens **(Fig. 81.3)** or are completely filled with homogeneous blood products **(50 in Fig. 81.4)**. Do you know why the fluid level in **Fig. 81.3** is almost vertical? The answer is found on page 125.

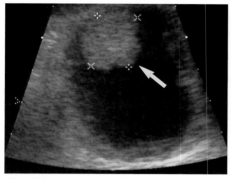

Fig. 81.1

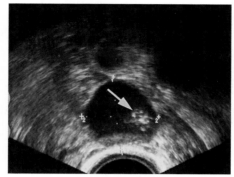

Fig. 81.2

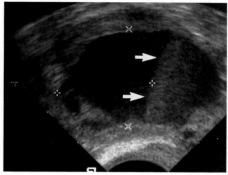

Fig. 81.3

Infertility Therapy

Measuring the hormone levels of an externally stimulated cycle neither allows one to definitively exclude hyperstimulated ovaries **(Fig. 81.5)** nor does it provide reliable information about the number of stimulated follicles **(93)**. Ultrasound monitoring of the number of growing Graafian follicles is indicated so that discontinuation of the hormone therapy can be considered where there are more than two stimulated follicles and the patient can take contraceptive measures if necessary.

About 5% of women have polycystic ovary syndrome (PCO), characterized by lack of typical follicular maturation. This is often due to adrenal hyperandrogenism. The typical features of PCO are multiple small cysts **(64)** arranged like a string of pearls primarily along the periphery of the ovary around a hyperechoic stroma **(91 in Fig. 81.6)**. Hormone therapy can help resolve such cases of undesired infertility.

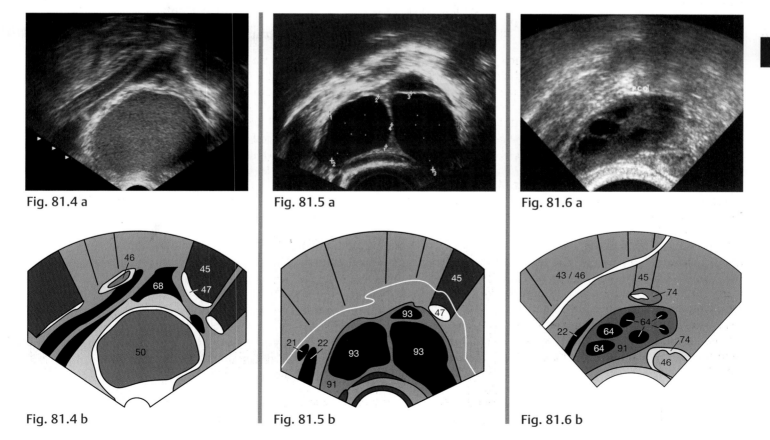

Fig. 81.4 a

Fig. 81.5 a

Fig. 81.6 a

Fig. 81.4 b

Fig. 81.5 b

Fig. 81.6 b

Pregnancy testing is not limited to measuring β-hCG in the maternal blood or urine. Additional ultrasound examinations can not only confirm the pregnancy, but also exclude an ectopic pregnancy. Ultrasound can also detect multiple pregnancy (**Figs. 83.3, 83.4**).

Ultrasound scans can detect an early intrauterine pregnancy (shown here is my first daughter, **Fig. 82.1**) once the chorionic cavity has reached a diameter of about 2–3 mm. This size is generally reached 14 days after conception, or 4 weeks and 3 days after the last menstruation.

The tiny chorionic cavity embedded in the hyperechoic endometrium (**78**) of the body of the uterus (**39**) enlarges at a rate of about 1.1 mm per day to become the gestational sac (**101**), in which the embryo (**95**) can later be identified (**Fig. 82.2**). Embryonic cardiac activities begin at a gestational age of 6 weeks with a heart rate of 80–90 beats per minute. Doppler sonography need not be routinely used to determine the cardiac rate as long as embryonic development is proceeding normally (see below).

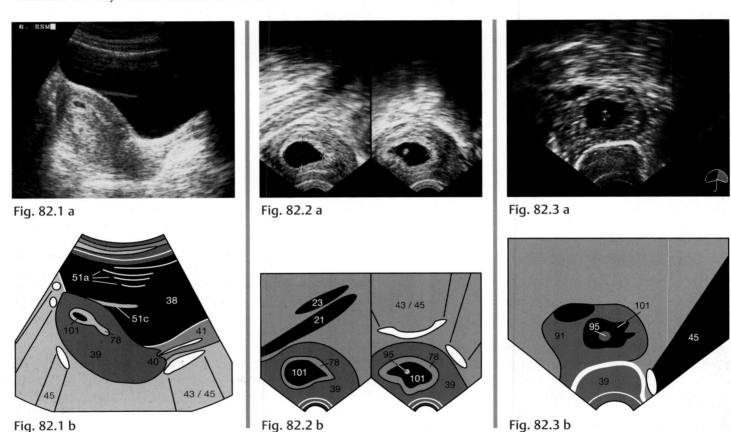

Fig. 82.1 a

Fig. 82.2 a

Fig. 82.3 a

Fig. 82.1 b

Fig. 82.2 b

Fig. 82.3 b

If an embryo is not identified in the chorionic cavity when expected, the first step is to verify gestational age. If a follow-up examination shows retarded growth of an empty chorionic cavity (see p. 84), a blighted ovum is present, which occurs in about 5% of all gestations.

Ectopic Pregnancy

In an ectopic pregnancy (**Fig. 82.3**), the gestational sac (**101**) is outside the uterus (**39**). Because of its severe consequences, this condition should not be missed.

Safety Threshold Discussion

According to the guidelines of the American Institute of Ultrasound in Medicine (AIUM), sound energies below 100 mW/cm^2 or 50 J/cm are safe. Because the energies delivered with B-scan imaging (black and white) are far lower, current knowledge indicates that neither relevant thermal injury to

tissue nor mutagenic effects are to be expected. This also applies to repeated ultrasound examinations during pregnancy. In this context, it is of interest to note that sound pulses are only emitted during a small fraction of the examination time, whereas most of the time is required to receive the reflected echoes.

The situation is different for color-coded Doppler and pulsed Doppler studies. These threshold values can be reached or exceeded during longer examinations. Although there has been no evidence to date of any damaging effect of ultrasound waves, any unnecessary color-coded Doppler studies should be avoided during the sensitive phase of organogenesis in the first trimester. References for these statements are available from the author.

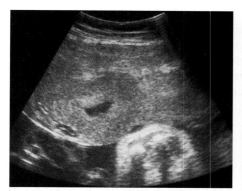

Fig. 83.1 a

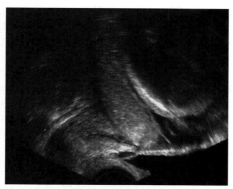

Fig. 83.2 a

The normal location of the placenta is near the fundus along the anterior or posterior uterine wall. In about 20% of cases, the placenta (94) will show one or more unilocular or multilocular cysts or lacunae (64), which usually have no functional significance (Fig. 83.1). However, an association with maternal diabetes or Rhesus incompatibility has been suggested.

The definitive location of the placenta cannot be reliably determined before the end of the second trimester. This is because the increasing expansion of the lower uterus can change what began as a placenta previa in early pregnancy to a normal or low-lying placenta (distance to internal os of the cervix < 5 cm).

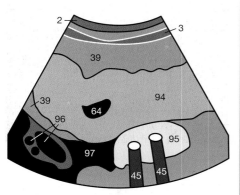

Fig. 83.1 b

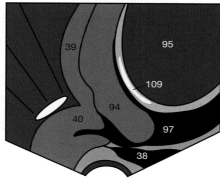

Fig. 83.2 b

Three types of placenta previa are distinguished: total placenta previa, which totally covers the internal os of the cervix (40); partial placenta previa, which partially covers the internal os (Fig. 83.2); and marginal placenta previa, which encroaches on the internal os. The evaluation of placental structure has become less important as placental and fetal perfusion can be evaluated with Doppler sonography.

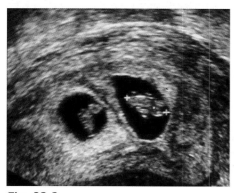

Fig. 83.3

Multiple Pregnancy

In multiple pregnancy, it must be determined whether the gestational sacs (95) share one placenta or are supplied by separate placentas (← in Fig. 83.4). Parents-to-be (and their obstetrician) like to know whether to expect twins (Fig. 83.3) or even triplets (Fig. 83.4). Some parents also want to know whether they are expecting a daughter (Fig. 83.5) or son (Fig. 83.6).

Gender Determination

Remember to reveal the gender of the fetus to the parents only when asked or if it has been previously requested. Above all, you should be certain of this determination. Early in pregnancy, it is possible to mistake the umbilical cord (↘) for a clitoris or (↖) penis, and the female labia for the scrotum (➡ in Figs. 83.5, 83.6).

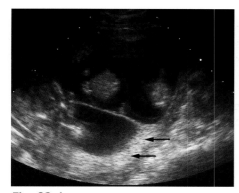

Fig. 83.4

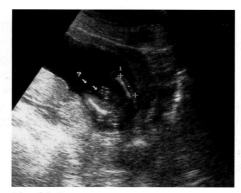

Fig. 83.5

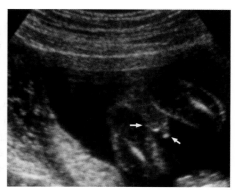

Fig. 83.6

With the help of biometric parameters, ultrasound can reveal early gestational growth disturbances and detect fetal malformations. The normal values of the subsequent measurements can be found as tables with median and percentile values (for the German population) on the internal back cover.

Chorionic Cavity Diameter (CCD)

The initially anechoic chorionic cavity (**101**) is surrounded by a hyperechoic rim of reactive endometrium (**78** in **Fig. 84.1**) and is visualized on ultrasound 14 days after conception. It should be detectable at serum hCG levels above 750–1000 U/L, otherwise an ectopic pregnancy must be excluded (see p. 82).

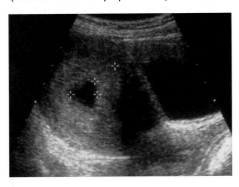

Fig. 84.1 a

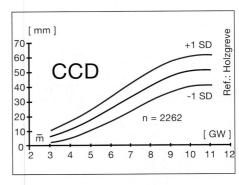

Fig. 84.1 b

Fig. 84.1 c

Yolk Sac Diameter (YSD)

The yolk sac is a hyperechoic ring structure with an anechoic center that increases to a size of about 5 mm at the 10th week of gestation. A yolk sac diameter under 3 mm or above 7 mm implies an increased risk of developmental anomalies. If the yolk sac is identified within the uterine cavity, an intrauterine pregnancy is established, as the yolk sac is an embryonal structure. **Fig. 84.2** shows a yolk sac (**102**) next to the spine (**35**) of an older embryo of a gestational age of 7 weeks and 6 days.

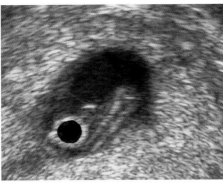

Fig. 84.2 a

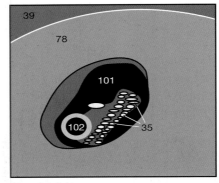

Fig. 84.2 b

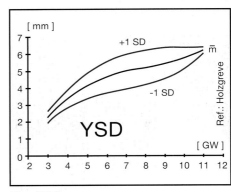

Fig. 84.2 c

Crown–Rump Length (CRL)

An intact embryo with a crown–rump length of 5 mm can be visualized beginning at a gestational age of 6 weeks and 3 days. At this time, the gestational sac measures 15 mm to 18 mm. Once there is a visible embryo (**95**), crown–rump length replaces measurement of chorionic cavity diameter as it allows more reliable determination of gestational age (within a few days) up to the 12th week of gestation (**Fig. 84.3**). Thereafter, biparietal skull diameter is more accurate (see p. 85).

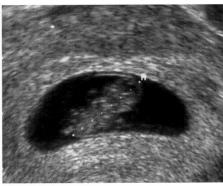

Fig. 84.3 a

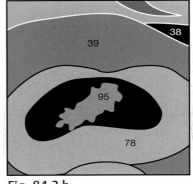

Fig. 84.3 b

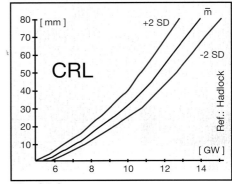

Fig. 84.3 c

Biparietal Skull Diameter (BPD)

Beginning with the 12th week of gestation, the biparietal skull diameter is a more practical and accurate measurement than crown–rump length. The choroid plexus **(104)** appears as a bilateral hyperechoic structure. To obtain exact and reproducible values, the biparietal skull diameter should always be measured on the continuous oval of the cranium **(105)** at the same reference level **(Fig. 85.1)**. It is important to measure along a line perpendicular to the midline echoes of the falx cerebri **(106)**, which is interrupted in its frontal third by the cavum of the septum lucidum. The imaging plane should not include the cerebellum or orbits as measurements at this level are too far caudal. Head circumference and fronto-occipital diameter can be measured at this same level. The normal values are found on the internal back cover and on the pocket-sized reference cards.

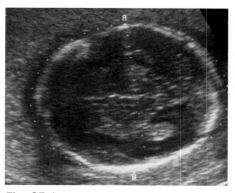

Fig. 85.1 a

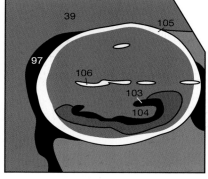

Fig. 85.1 b

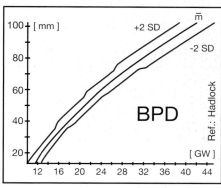

Fig. 85.1 c

Femur Length (FL)

Measuring the ossified femoral diaphysis **(107)** is relatively easy. The long axis of the upper thigh **(108)** should be in a transverse position, parallel to the surface axis of the transducer **(Fig. 85.2)**. Measurements of other tubular bones are obtained only for clarification when the femoral length falls outside the normal range or when serial measurements cross the percentiles, i.e., when growth retardation or malformation must be excluded.

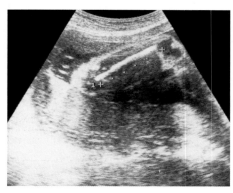

Fig. 85.2 a

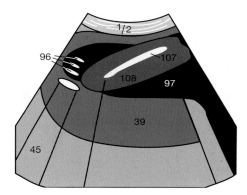

Fig. 85.2 b

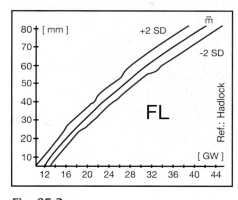

Fig. 85.2 c

Abdominal Circumference (AC)

The abdominal circumference **(Fig. 85.3)** is measured at the level of the liver **(9)**, wherever possible visualizing the posterior third of the umbilical and portal veins **(11)** as well. The sectioned ribs should appear symmetric, indicating the image has not been obtained in an oblique plane.

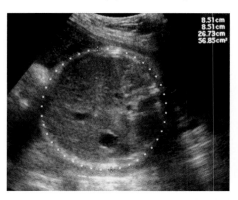

Fig. 85.3 a

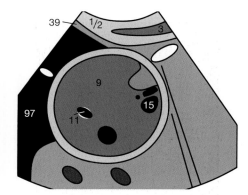

Fig. 85.3 b

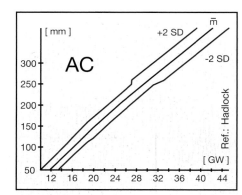

Fig. 85.3 c

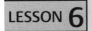

Cerebellum

The cerebellum **(110)** is visualized on a transverse section through the posterior cranial fossa **(Fig. 86.1)**. There should be a physiologic posterior indentation (◀). Its absence ("banana sign") suggests caudal displacement of the cerebellum toward the spinal canal **(Fig. 86.2)** as in spina bifida.

The cranial vault **(105)** can lose its typical oval shape on transverse cerebral sections for the same reason. It then resembles a sliced lemon ("lemon sign") with scalloping (↙) of the parietal bones bilaterally **(Fig. 86.3)**. Here, the hyperechoic choroid plexus **(104)** is also visualized.

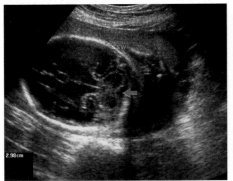

Fig. 86.1 a

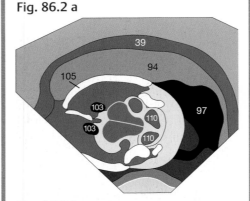

Fig. 86.2 a

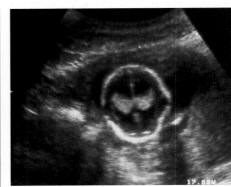

Fig. 86.3 a

Fig. 86.1 b

Fig. 86.2 b

Fig. 86.3 b

CSF Spaces

The choroid plexus can occasionally contain small unilateral cysts (◣ in **Fig. 86.4**). Although they usually lack any clinical significance, bilateral cysts have been associated with trisomy 18 and, rarely, with renal and cardiac malformations. Hydrocephalus **(Fig. 86.5)** such as in aqueductal stenosis or spina bifida is associated with other intracellular and extracellular malformations in 70–90% of all cases.

The reference value for a hydrocephalus is a ventricle-hemisphere ratio exceeding 0.5 after the 20th week of gestation. A distinction is made between the ratio of the anterior horn diameter to the hemispheric diameter and that of the occipital horn diameter to the hemispheric diameter, which is slightly higher **(Fig. 86.6b)**. Obtaining this measurement can be difficult because often the lateral ventricular wall is not sharply demarcated from the cerebral parenchyma **(Fig. 86.6a)**.

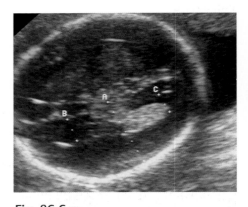

Fig. 86.6 a

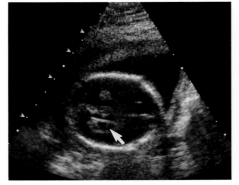

Fig. 86.4

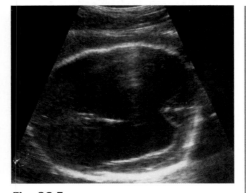

Fig. 86.5

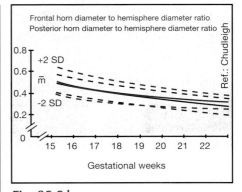

Fig. 86.6 b

Spinal Anatomy

The spine (35) is scanned in the sagittal plane (**Fig. 87.1**), visualized in the coronal plane (**Fig. 87.2**), and subsequently scanned craniocaudally over its entire length so that the examiner can see any interruption in the chain of the spinous processes. In the axial plane (**Fig. 87.3**), it is important that the three ossification centers (35) in each segment form a close triangle. The fetal aorta (15) lies anterior to the spine.

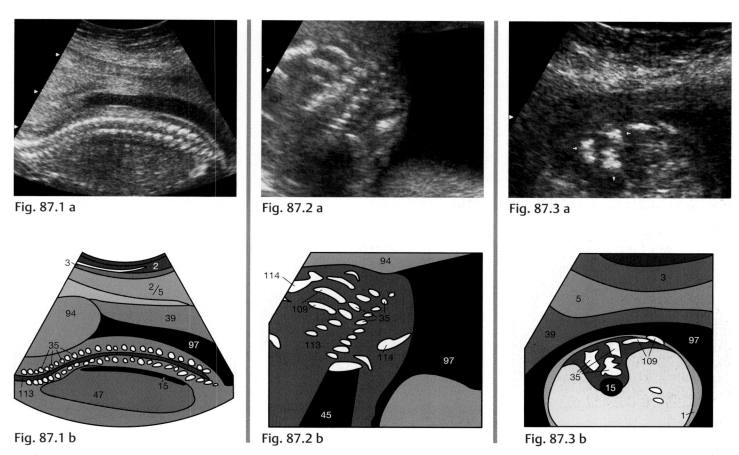

Fig. 87.1 a   Fig. 87.2 a   Fig. 87.3 a

Fig. 87.1 b   Fig. 87.2 b   Fig. 87.3 b

Spina Bifida

Spina bifida is a malformation due to incomplete fusion of the neural tube combined with variable defects of the vertebral arches. Spina bifida (**Fig. 87.4**) widens the distance between the two posterior ossification centers (✖ ✖). Measuring the maternal serum levels of alpha feto-protein alone is diagnostic only for spina bifida cystica (spina bifida aperta). It does not detect spina bifida occulta, where there is no protrusion of the spinal cord.

Indirect cerebral signs of a spina bifida that are detectable in the fetal cranium include the "banana" and "lemon" signs shown on page 86.

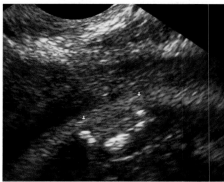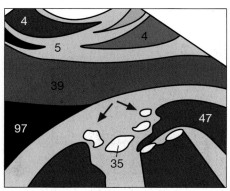

Fig. 87.4 a   Fig. 87.4 b

Facial Bones

The face is usually examined in the transverse and coronal planes for a decreased interocular distance (hypotelorism) or increased interocular distance (hypertelorism). It is examined in the sagittal plane for an unusual profile. Cleft lip and palate usually occurs at a lateral location. It is most easily detected in the coronal plane as an interrupted hyperechoic upper lip. Normally the upper lip (➡, ➘) is visualized as a continuous structure **(Fig. 88.1)**.

Nuchal Translucency (NT)

Edema of the cervical subcutaneous tissue (nuchal translucency) detected between the 10th and 14th weeks of gestation (or at a crown–rump length between 38 and 84 mm) and exceeding 3 mm in width suggests impaired lymphatic drainage. As many as one-third of these cases are associated with chromosomal abnormalities such as chromosome XO syndrome (Turner syndrome), trisomy 21 (Down syndrome), and trisomy 18.

To distinguish the nuchal skin from amnion that is merely in close contact with the fetal skin, it is important to wait for spontaneous fetal activity. Nuchal skin visualized tangentially can also mimic a double contour (⬇ in **Fig. 88.2**), although this invariably

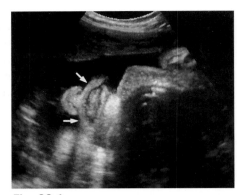

Fig. 88.1

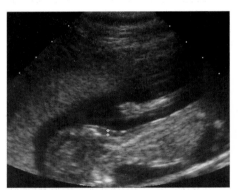

Fig. 88.2 a

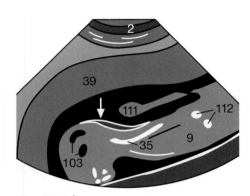

Fig. 88.2 b

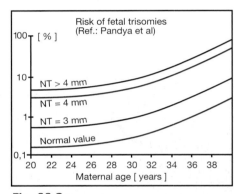

Fig. 88.2 c

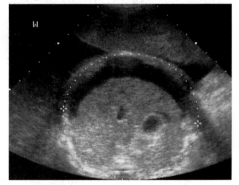

Fig. 88.3 a

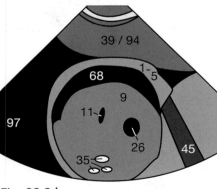

Fig. 88.3 b

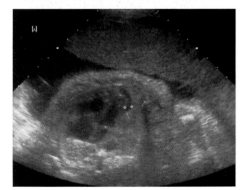

Fig. 88.4 a

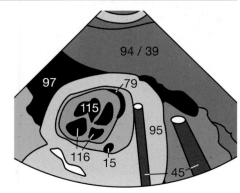

Fig. 88.4 b

measures less than 3 mm. The risk of a chromosomal abnormality increases with the width of the nuchal translucency and maternal age **(Fig. 88.2c)**.

Hydrops Fetalis

Several conditions lead to increased accumulation of fluid in serous cavities and in the placenta. It can be caused by heart failure, anemia due to infection, congenital fetal anemia, Rhesus incompatibility, chromosomal abnormalities, or metabolic disorders.

In monozygotic twins, hydrops fetalis of one twin is caused by twin-to-twin transfusion through arteriovenous shunts. Aside from ascites (**68** in **Fig. 88.3**) and pleural or pericardial effusion (**79** in **Fig. 88.4**), ultrasound may also demonstrate generalized cutaneous edema.

Checklist for Hydrops Fetalis

- Ascites
- Pleural effusions
- Pericardial effusions
- Generalized cutaneous edema

The cardiovascular system is the first functioning system of the embryo. Cardiac contractions are visible beginning in the 6th week of gestation. Absent cardiac contractions and arrested growth of the gestational sac, which at this point has often become indistinctly demarcated, suggest a missed abortion, which generally requires dilatation and curettage.

Doppler and color-coded Doppler sonography should be avoided wherever possible because of their high sound intensities (see p. 82). They should only be applied in cases of suspected growth retardation or cardiac malformation.

Cardiac Anatomy

First, one should verify the location of the heart. At the level of the four-chamber view, one-third of the heart lies to the right of an imaginary line between the spine and the anterior chest wall, and two-thirds are to the left of this line. The sagittal plane (Fig. 89.1) should pass through the aortic arch (15) and origins of the supra-aortic branches, which include the brachiocephalic trunk (117), the left common carotid artery (82), and the left subclavian artery (123). In addition to the

valves, one must also identify the atria (116) and ventricles (115) on the four-chamber view (Fig. 89.2) and exclude a ventricular or atrial septal defect.

By slightly tilting the transducer, the inflow tract of the mitral valve (118) and the outflow tract of the left ventricle over the aortic valve (119) come into view on the so-called "five-chamber" view (Fig. 89.3).

Diagnosis of Congenital Cardiac Shunts

A ventricular septal defect in the membranous part of the interventricular septum is best seen on the five-chamber view. However, definitive exclusion of small atrial or ventricular septal defects or cardiovascular shunts requires supplementary color-coded echocardiography performed by an experienced examiner.

Even transposition of the great vessels can be overlooked on the four-chamber view. It is therefore essential to examine not only the crossing of the outflow tracts, but also the aortic and pulmonary valves on the short axis view.

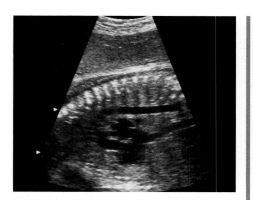

Fig. 89.1 a

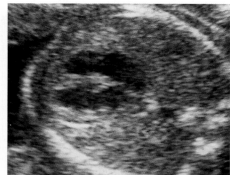

Fig. 89.2 a

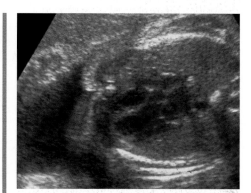

Fig. 89.3 a

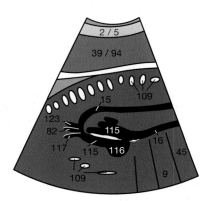

Fig. 89.1 b

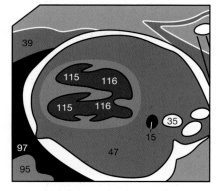

Fig. 89.2 b

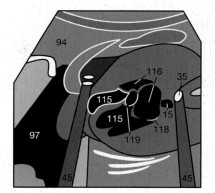

Fig. 89.3 b

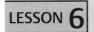
Gastrointestinal Tract

When evaluating the gastrointestinal tract, the examiner must be alert to the "double bubble" sign, which suggests duodenal atresia or stenosis. Two adjacent fluid-filled (anechoic) bubbles can represent the stomach and duodenal segment proximal to the stenosis.

The diagnosis should be confirmed in two planes to avoid a false-positive diagnosis mimicked by a tangentially visualized stomach that is sectioned by the sound beam twice.

Umbilical Hernia and Omphalocele

Bear in mind that herniation of the fetal bowel (120) through the anterior abdominal wall (Fig. 90.1) next to the umbilical vessels (96) is physiologic until the 11th week of gestation. This must not be mistaken for a true omphalocele (a pathologic extrusion of abdominal organs).

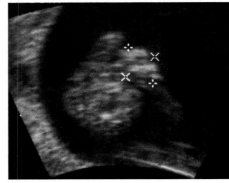

Fig. 90.1 a

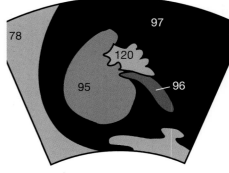

Fig. 90.1 b

Kidneys

Beginning in the 15th week of gestation, renal malformations are often indirectly detectable as insufficient amniotic fluid (oligohydramnios), absence of amniotic fluid, or an empty bladder. At this stage of fetal development, the amniotic fluid represents renal urinary excretion. The relatively hypoechoic medullary pyramids (30) and the anechoic renal pelvis (31) are already identifiable on the longitudinal view (Fig. 90.2) of the normal renal parenchyma (29). An overview of the intrauterine growth of the kidneys is shown in Fig. 90.2c.

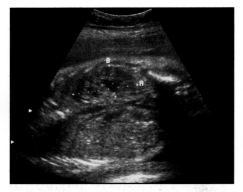

Fig. 90.2 a

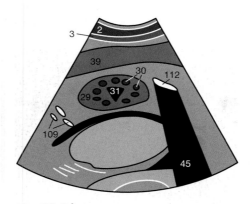

Fig. 90.2 b

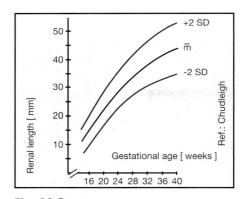

Fig. 90.2 c

Fetal urinary obstruction caused by stenosis of the ureteropelvic junction is best detected on a transverse view of the kidneys (Fig. 90.3) by comparing both sides. Cystic renal diseases manifest themselves either only in adulthood (Potter type III) or on prenatal ultrasound scans as multicystic (Potter type II) or microcystic hyperechoic (Potter type I) kidneys.

Potter type III disease can also be detected on prenatal scans as diffusely increased renal echogenicity in the presence of a normal amount of amniotic fluid and a full bladder.

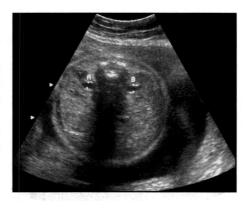

Fig. 90.3 a

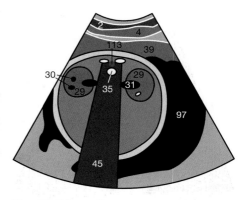

Fig. 90.3 b

Hands

In the second and third trimesters, the hands (**Fig. 91.1**) are examined to verify completeness of the phalangeal ossification centers **(121)** and metacarpal bones **(122)**. This examination can not only exclude syndactyly in the setting of other malformation syndromes, it can also detect polydactyly with supernumerary phalanges (see below).

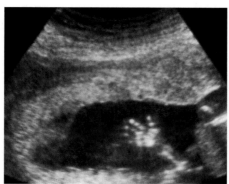

Fig. 91.1 a

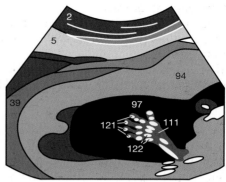

Fig. 91.1 b

Feet

Where the intrauterine mobility of the fetus and the experience of the examiner allow it, the feet can be so clearly visualized (**Fig. 91.2**) that it is possible to count the metatarsals **(122)** and toes **(121)**. **Fig. 91.3** shows hexadactyly (6 toes). Polydactyly is occasionally associated with shortened ribs, a bell-shaped thorax, and secondary pulmonary hypoplasia.

Clubfoot

Do not forget to rule out a clubfoot deformity (**Fig. 91.4**), which includes not only a thickened foot but also positional anomalies and curved or shortened tubular bones.

Dysplastic enchondral ossification in the setting of achondroplasia is often only detected in the third trimester. Tubular bones appear shortened in comparison with the disproportionately large head.

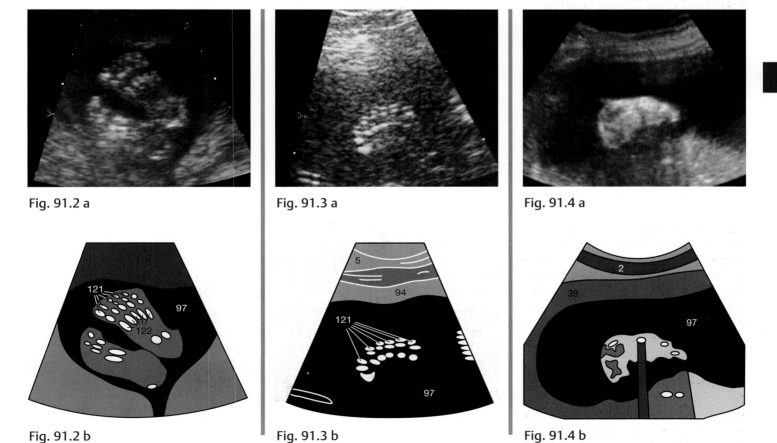

Fig. 91.2 a

Fig. 91.3 a

Fig. 91.4 a

Fig. 91.2 b

Fig. 91.3 b

Fig. 91.4 b

To complete this chapter, we again offer you the opportunity to test which details you have remembered and where your knowledge is still patchy. The answers to quiz questions 1 through 6 can be found on the preceding pages, while the answer to the image question (no. 7) is on page 124 at the end of the book.

1. On page 81, you were asked why a fluid level in a hemorrhagic endometrial cyst was vertical on the ultrasound image. Do you know the answer? If not, please review the description of the sagittal imaging planes on endovaginal ultrasound on p. 77.

2. An 18-year-old male patient presents with severe pain in the left scrotum, which began about three hours earlier and radiates into the left groin. What are the main causes you must consider in a differential diagnosis? How much time do you have to establish the diagnosis? What sonographic methods do you plan to use?

3. How do you recognize imminent ovulation on an ultrasound scan? What should change after the ovulation? How many days after the last menstruation or conception it is possible to document nidation on endovaginal ultrasound?

4. List six biometric parameters (measurements of fetal organ sizes obtained during prenatal care) next to this text. Next to each, write the first and last weeks of gestation within which the respective measurements are meaningful. When is one parameter replaced by another?

5. What are the direct and indirect sonographic criteria of spina bifida? Is serologic examination of the mother sufficient? Why or why not?

6. What renal malformations are detectable in the fetus? Please list at least three sonographic criteria of these malformations.

7. A 58-year-old female patient is referred to you for a routine gynecologic examination. The patient had her menopause at age 52 years and has not taken any hormone medications within the last 5 years. You perform an endovaginal ultrasound examination and detect the findings shown in **Fig. 92.1**. The transverse diameter of the endometrium is 18 mm. What is your tentative diagnosis and what further steps would you take?

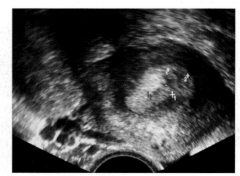

Fig. 92.1

Optimal conditions for examining newborns and infants include not only a quiet environment free of any hectic activity, a prewarmed gel, and a heat lamp over the examination table, but also the presence of a person emotionally close to the child.

The examination is performed through the anterior fontanel (135 in Fig. 93.1) until it closes at the age of about 1½ years. The size of the acoustic window steadily decreases with age, making it increasingly difficult to visualize lateral and peripheral cerebral structures, even with maximal tilting of the transducer.

The transducers that have proven most useful are multifrequency sector transducers (Fig. 93.1c) with a small contact coupling area and a center frequency of about 3.0 MHz for infants, 5.0 MHz for ages 6–8 months, or 7.5 MHz for preterm and term newborns. Transducers are now available that combine the good near-field resolution of linear transducers with a beam that diverges in the deeper layers. This makes it possible to visualize a wider segment of the brain (Fig. 93.1c).

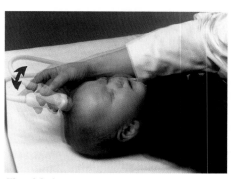

Fig. 93.1 a

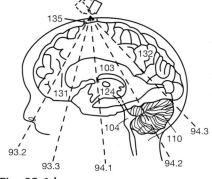

Fig. 93.1 b

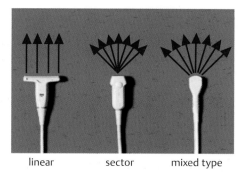

linear   sector   mixed type

Fig. 93.1 c

The skull is scanned in the coronal and sagittal planes (see p. 86) with a slow and continuous sweep of the transducer (Fig. 93.1a, b). The examination passes through and documents five standard coronal planes. One begins anteriorly (Fig. 93.2) and inspects the periventricular white matter (131), which is more hyperechoic than the overlying cortex (132). The transducer rests on the superior sagittal sinus (136).

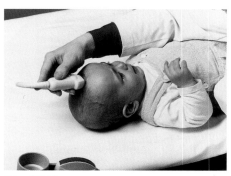

Fig. 93.2 a

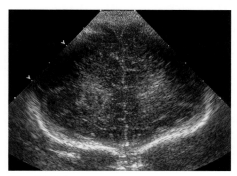

Fig. 93.2 b

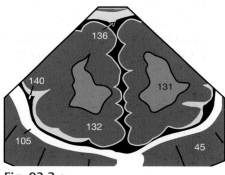

Fig. 93.2 c

The plane immediately posterior to the first one (Fig. 93.3) intersects the anterior horns of both lateral ventricles (103), which in this plane should not contain any hyperechoic choroid plexus. Slight ventricular asymmetry can still be physiologic or can be due to oblique sectioning. The shape of the hyperechoic Sylvian fissure (134) resembles a Y rotated 90° (see Fig. 94.1c).

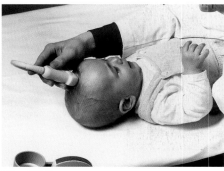

Fig. 93.3 a

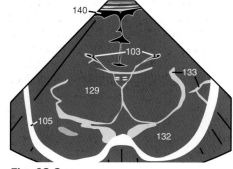

Fig. 93.3 b

Fig. 93.3 c

The transducer is now moved posteriorly to the next imaging plane to document the communication between the lateral ventricles (103) and the third ventricle (124) through the interventricular foramen of Monro (144 in Fig. 94.1). In addition to anechoic cerebrospinal fluid, the hyperechoic choroid plexus (104) is visualized in the lumen of this ventricular communication. This hyperechoic choroid plexus must not be mistaken for an intraventricular hemorrhage, which would be equally hyperechoic.

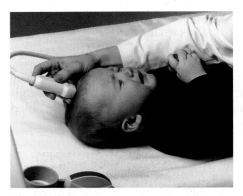

Fig. 94.1 a

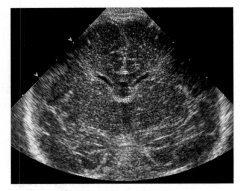

Fig. 94.1 b

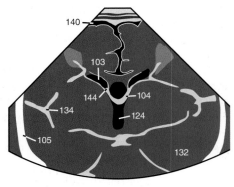

Fig. 94.1 c

Tilting the transducer further anteriorly (Fig. 94.2a) causes the sound waves to propagate further occipitally. This visualizes the curved bodies of both lateral ventricles, which merge with the temporal horns (Fig. 94.2b). Here it is also easy to determine the width of the lateral ventricles (103) and thickness of the choroid plexus (104), which is normally smoothly demarcated. The thalamus, internal capsule, and putamen are located medially.

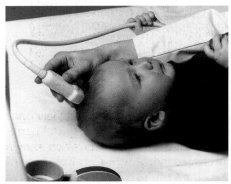

Fig. 94.2 a

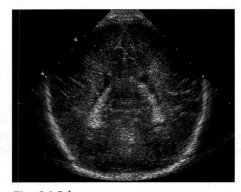

Fig. 94.2 b

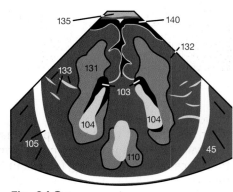

Fig. 94.2 c

Placing the transducer at an extreme angle (Fig. 94.3a) visualizes the somewhat ill-defined and hyperechoic occipital white matter (131 in Fig. 94.3b), which surrounds the ventricle in a pattern resembling a butterfly. Note the many sulci (133) that traverse the cortex as hyperechoic lines because of their rich vascularity and connective tissue. The normal widths of the CSF spaces are shown on the next page.

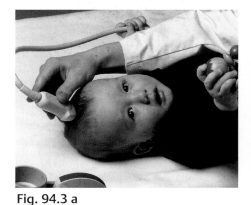

Fig. 94.3 a

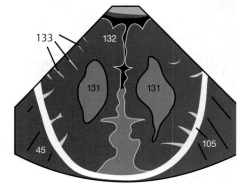

Fig. 94.3 b

Fig. 94.3 c

CSF Spaces

Additional images of the subarachnoid space and other superficial structures are obtained with a linear transducer of 5.0 to 7.5 MHz to achieve adequate resolution **(Fig. 95.1)**. In the neonate, the normal width of the anterior horns **(103)** measured from the midline complex of the falx cerebri **(106)** to the lateral ventricular wall should not exceed 13 mm. The measurements are made at the level of the foramen of Monro **(144)** or third ventricle **(124)**. The width of the third ventricle should not exceed 10 mm.

The subarachnoid space is measured at three levels. The interhemispheric fissure **(146)**, measured at the level of two opposite sulci, has a maximum width of 6 mm in the neonate. Sinocortical width **(147,** < 3 mm) and craniocortical width

CSF Spaces in the Newborn		
SCW	(Sinocortical width)	< 3 mm
CCW	(Craniocortical width)	< 4 mm
IHW	(Interhemispheric width)	< 6 mm
LVW	(Lateral ventricle width, anterior horn)	< 13 mm
3rd VW	(Width of third ventricle)	< 10 mm

(148, < 4 mm) are determined to exclude cerebral atrophy (with expansion of the subarachnoid space) or noncommunicating hydrocephalus (with narrowing of the subarachnoid space).

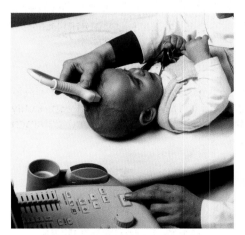

Fig. 95.1 a

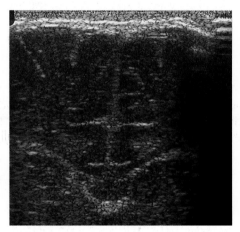

Fig. 95.1 b

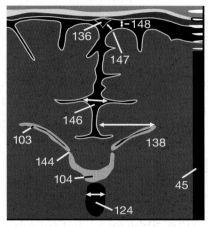

Fig. 95.1 c

Sagittal Plane

After the scans in the coronal plane have been completed, sagittal plane imaging is then performed by rotating the transducer 90° and sweeping from right to left on the anterior fontanel **(Fig. 95.2a)**. It is recommended that each examiner establish a standard examination sequence. This will minimize the risk of confusing right and left.

For example, one can make it a habit to systematically scan first the left hemisphere, then the median plane, then the

right hemisphere for pathologic changes. Please review once more the normal topographic anatomy of the sagittal hemispheric sections from a midline transducer position shown in **Fig. 95.2c**. It is important to verify normal morphology of the corpus callosum **(126)** and the overlying cingulate gyrus **(130)**. The cerebellum **(110)** is visualized as a hyperechoic structure posterior to the pons **(145)** in the posterior cranial fossa (see **Fig. 96.2**).

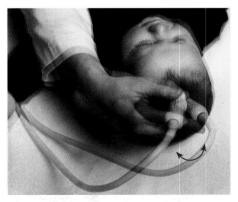

Fig. 95.2 a

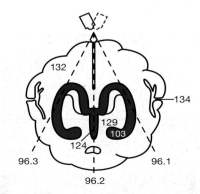

Fig. 95.2 b

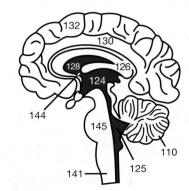

Fig. 95.2 c

P

Sagittal Planes

The thalamus (129) lies at the center of the laterally oblique imaging planes (Figs. 96.1 and 96.3). The anechoic CSF in the lateral ventricle (103) is above the thalamus and contains the hyperechoic choroid plexus (104), whose contour should be smooth without local bulging. This must be distinguished from a choroid plexus hemorrhage (see p. 98). Where the corpus callosum (126) is normally developed, the cerebral sulci (133) of the parietal and occipital lobes do not extend to the lateral ventricles, but are interrupted by the cingulate gyrus (130).

Fig. 96.1 shows an oblique sagittal section through the left lateral ventricle. A midline section including the pons (145), hyperechoic cerebellum (110), and fourth ventricle (125) is shown in Fig. 96.2.

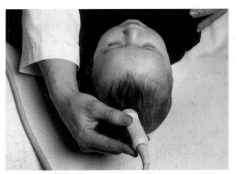

Fig. 96.1 a

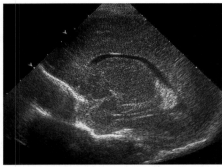

Fig. 96.1 b

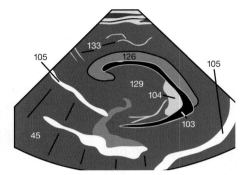

Fig. 96.1 c

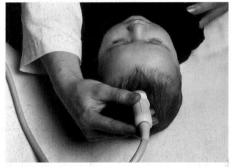

Fig. 96.2 a

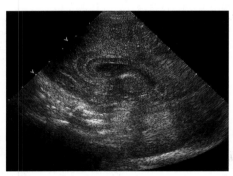

Fig. 96.2 b

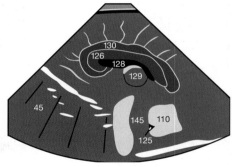

Fig. 96.2 c

Choroid Plexus Cysts

Small unilateral choroid plexus cysts (64) represent normal variants (Fig. 96.3). These are most probably the result of small prenatal hemorrhages, although prenatal viral infections have been discussed as a possible cause. If the cyst is small and does not impair the CSF circulation, it generally has no clinical consequence. Only larger parenchymal defects that are isoechoic to CSF (porencephaly) suggest areas of hemorrhage resorption or cerebral malformations.

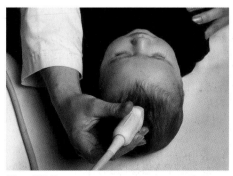

Fig. 96.3 a

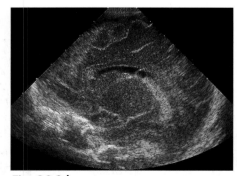

Fig. 96.3 b

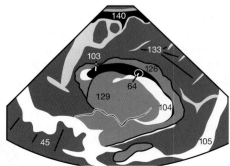

Fig. 96.3 c

Preterm Newborns

The normal cerebral sulci can be totally absent in preterm newborns delivered around the 28th week of gestation. Cerebral gyration is usually less well developed on ultrasound scans of preterm newborns than in term newborns. However, this is not necessarily indicative of a genuine maturation disturbance. Accordingly, the CSF spaces in a preterm newborn are more capacious and occasionally asymmetric (**Fig. 97.2**).

The corpus callosum is often incompletely developed in preterm newborns as well. It then appears as a thin hypoechoic line in the coronal plane, usually just above the cavum of the septum pellucidum. These physiologic signs of immaturity will have to be monitored on follow-up studies to distinguish them from impaired CSF flow or genuine hypoplasia or agenesis of the corpus callosum (**Fig. 97.3**).

Cavum of the Septum Pellucidum

Incomplete fusion of the septum pellucidum between the anterior horns leads to a CSF-filled cavum of the septum pellucidum (**128**). This is usually obliterated within the first few months of life but persists into adulthood in about 20% of cases (**Fig. 97.1**). A slitlike CSF-filled space in a more occipital location is referred to as a cavum vergae.

Slight asymmetry of the lateral ventricles (**103**) is another normal variant that is not necessarily indicative of impaired CSF flow. **Fig. 97.2** shows a wide anechoic CSF space lateral to the choroid plexus (**104**) on the left, but not on the right (the coronal images are viewed from the front so that the hemispheres are reversed).

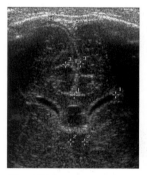

Fig. 97.1 a

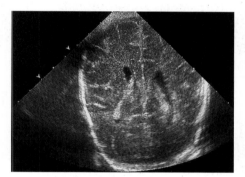

Fig. 97.2 a

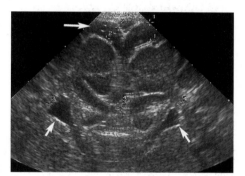

Fig. 97.3 a

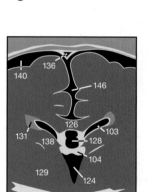

Fig. 97.1 b

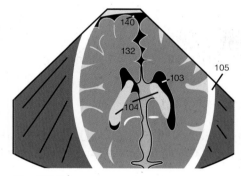

Fig. 97.2 b

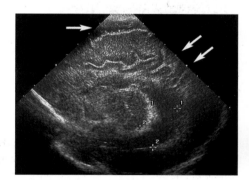

Fig. 97.3 b

Agenesis of the Corpus Callosum

Many developmental disorders, syndromes, and metabolic disorders involve the corpus callosum, and involvement may also be secondary to hypoxia or infection. The spectrum of callosal abnormalities ranges from partial to complete absence (agenesis) of the corpus callosum. In the coronal plane (**Fig. 97.3a**), agenesis of the corpus callosum leads to a "steer horn" appearance of both anterior horns (➚ ➘), which are farther apart and farther lateral than normal.

In the sagittal plane (**Fig. 97.3b**), the cingulate gyrus is absent (see **Fig. 96.1**) so that the gyri of the cerebral hemispheres extend to the lateral ventricles (➘ ➘). This makes it easy to detect even partial agenesis of the corpus callosum. The example in **Fig. 97.3** shows prominent lateral ventricles and a prominent subarachnoid space (➡) in the setting of diffuse cerebral atrophy (compare **Fig. 96.1**).

Pathophysiology

The ventricles are lined by an epithelium known as the ependyma. The subependymal tissue layer proliferates between the 24th and 32nd weeks of gestation and becomes richly vascularized. During this time, this germinal matrix is very sensitive to fluctuations in blood pressure as the mechanism for regulating intracerebral blood flow is not yet developed.

As a result, fetal cerebral hemorrhage very often occurs in the subependymal region or in the region of the choroid plexus. Four grades of cerebral hemorrhage are distinguished according to severity, as shown in the table to the right.

Cerebral Hemorrhage: Grading	
Grade 1	Isolated subependymal hemorrhage
Grade 2	Subependymal hemorrhage with ventricular extension (involving less than 50% of the ventricular lumen) without ventricular dilation
Grade 3	Intraventricular hemorrhage (involving more than 50% of the lumen) and ventricular dilation
Grade 4	Additional extension into the cerebral parenchyma

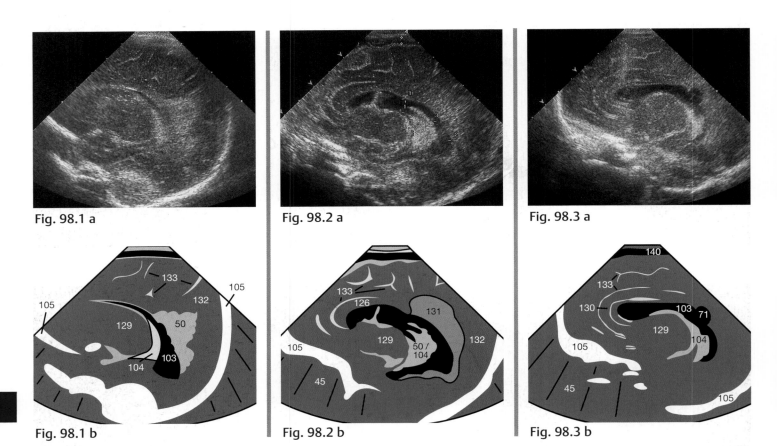

Fig. 98.1 a

Fig. 98.2 a

Fig. 98.3 a

Fig. 98.1 b

Fig. 98.2 b

Fig. 98.3 b

Ultrasound Morphology

Acute hemorrhage (50) is hyperechoic compared with the adjacent cerebral parenchyma (132) and usually located in the vicinity of the ventricles (Fig. 98.1) for the reasons outlined above. An irregularly shaped or bulging choroid plexus (104) suggests a hemorrhage (50) in the plexus (Fig. 98.2).

An earlier intrauterine hemorrhage that has been resorbed leaves behind CSF-filled parenchymal defects (71) that can be mistaken for dilation of a lateral ventricle (103 in Fig. 98.3). The differential diagnosis between a periventricular parenchymal defect and genuine hydrocephalus will be discussed on the next page.

P

Hydrocephalus

Obstructive (noncommunicating) hydrocephalus **(Fig. 99.1)** is usually caused by posthemorrhagic subarachnoid adhesions that obstruct the free flow of cerebrospinal fluid out of the ventricular system. Less frequent causes include compression of CSF channels by an aneurysm of the vein of Galen, a biconvex cyst of the septum pellucidum (see cavum of the septum pellucidum, **Fig. 97.1**) obstructing the foramen of Monro, or aqueduct stenosis. Isolated dilation of the fourth ventricle occurs where aqueduct stenosis is accompanied by obstruction of the foramina of Luschka and Magendie.

The resulting increase in intraventricular pressure initially produces rounded and distended temporal horns because here the pressure of the surrounding cerebral parenchyma is lowest. Thickening and dilation of the entire lateral ventricles **(Fig. 99.1)** only occurs later and is accompanied by narrowing of the subarachnoid space. The resulting increase in pressure must be slowly relieved by a diversionary CSF shunt (↖ in **Fig. 99.2**).

In chronic hydrocephalus, excessively rapid decompression could place strain on the external cerebral vessels (with risk of hemorrhage). After a CSF shunt has been placed, follow-up examinations are indicated to monitor the position of the shunt and exclude malfunction.

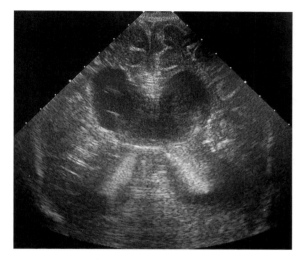

Fig. 99.1

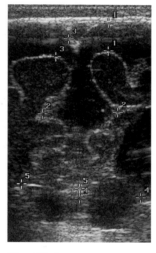

Fig. 99.3 a

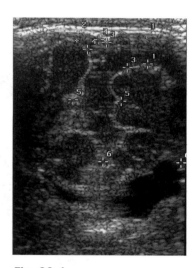

Fig. 99.4 a

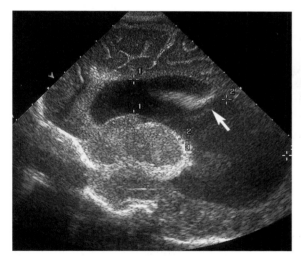

Fig. 99.2

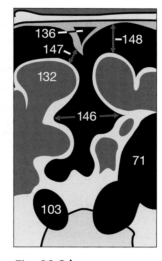

Fig. 99.3 b

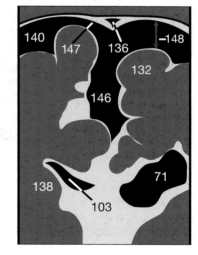

Fig. 99.4 b

Cerebral Atrophy

The width of the subarachnoid space can differentiate obstructive hydrocephalus from an enlarged ventricular system due to cerebral atrophy. Here, a linear transducer is used because of its better near-field resolution. **Fig. 99.3** shows significant widening of all CSF spaces in diffuse cerebral atrophy involving both hemispheres (compare to **Fig. 95.1**). Note the unusually good visualization of the superior sagittal sinus (136). Unilateral parenchymal defects (71) result in widening of the ipsilateral subarachnoid space (148) in comparison with the contralateral side (**Fig. 99.4**). Additionally, the superficial cerebral sulci are more prominent in cerebral atrophy, whereas they tend to be effaced in obstructive hydrocephalus.

Monitoring the Shunt in Hydrocephalus

Where ultrasound findings such as progressive ventricular enlargement suggest malfunction of the CSF shunt, the examiner should evaluate not only the intraventricular position of the shunt tip (see **Fig. 99.2**) but also the entire length of the shunt catheter.

The adjacent radiographs show a disconnected (✔) shunt **(Fig. 100.1a)** and the results of shunt revision **(Fig. 100.1b)** in a child with a ventriculoperitoneal shunt. On the second radiograph, the catheter has been reconnected to the coupling. Shunts occasionally need to be replaced or revised after several years as the child grows taller.

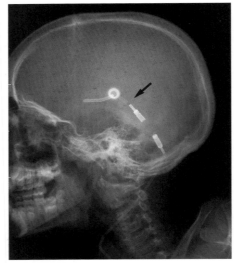

Fig. 100.1 a

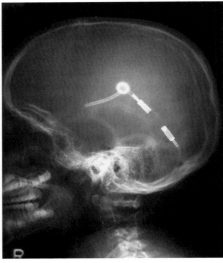

Fig. 100.1 b

Spinal Canal

In infants, the conus medullaris **(142)** of the spinal cord **(141)** is visualized on a posteroanterior scan of the prone patient using a 5.0 to 7.5 MHz transducer **(Fig. 100.2)**. The spinal cord is demarcated from the anechoic spinal CSF space **(140)** by the delicate hyperechoic line of the pia mater. The hyperechoic double line in the center of the cord is not the central canal but the interface between the white commissure and the anterior median fissure.

The roots of the cauda equina **(143)** extend caudally and are visualized as a hyperechoic structure around the conus medullaris (✖), which should not extend below the L2-L3 disk space in the newborn.

Anatomic landmarks: The beginning of the sacrum can be identified by its fused S1 vertebra, which is the first structure to protrude posteriorly (toward the transducer) from the straight line of the vertebrae.

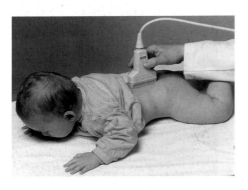

Fig. 100.2 a

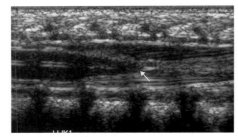

Fig. 100.2 b

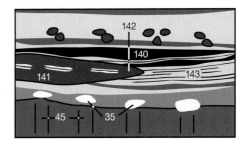

Fig. 100.2 c

The progressive ossification of the vertebral arches makes visualization of the spinal cord increasingly difficult on ultrasound images, and gradually requires the use of magnetic resonance imaging (MRI). It is important to verify unrestricted mobility of the spinal cord with respiration and pulse. This can be documented on M-mode studies.

Absent pulsation, distortion, or a low conus medullaris and fixation of the cord to the spinal canal suggest a tethered cord syndrome, which is often caused by an intraspinal lipoma or epidermoid cyst. A tethered cord can also occur from fixation of neural structures as a result of postsurgical scarring.

Anatomy

The thyroid gland is examined with a 7.5 MHz linear trans-ducer. The patient is positioned with the head slightly extend-ed. The thyroid gland is systematically scanned in successive transverse planes moving in a craniocaudal direction (**Fig. 101.1a**). Next, sagittal images are obtained through each thyroid lobe (**Fig. 101.1b**). The midline acoustic shadow of the trachea (**84**) and, farther laterally, the anechoic cross sec-tions of the carotid artery (**82**) and jugular vein (**83**) provide anatomic landmarks for the transverse images. The thyroid parenchyma (**81**) lies between these vessels and the trachea. A thin parenchymal band (isthmus) anterior to the trachea connects the two lobes of the thyroid (**Fig. 101.2**). The carotid artery (**82**) usually lies in a posteromedial location, and is round and incompressible in the transverse plane. The jugular vein (**83**) is farther anterolateral. It exhibits a typical biphasic venous pulse and is compressible when gentle pressure is applied to the transducer.

When in doubt about the identity of any of the vascular structures, the examiner can ask the patient to briefly press with the mouth closed. The resulting venous congestion distends the jugular vein, which usually provides a clear a natomic landmark. The normal thyroid parenchyma is slightly more hyperechoic (brighter) than the sternohyoid (**89**) and sternothyroid (**90**) muscles anterior to it and the sternocleido-mastoid (**85**) muscle farther lateral (**Fig. 101.2**).

Volumetric Measurements

To determine the volume of the thyroid gland, the maximum transverse and sagittal (anteroposterior) diameters of each lobe are measured on transverse sections. These values are multiplied by the craniocaudal length as measured on the sag-ittal section and the product is multiplied by 0.5. The result corresponds to the volume of each lateral lobe (in mL), with a margin of error of approximately 10%. The volume of both lobes should be < 25 mL in men and < 18 mL in women (see table on p. 103).

Small cysts (**64**) in the thyroid gland (**81**) may not cause any distal acoustic enhancement (**Fig. 101.3b**) and must be dif-ferentiated from hypoechoic nodules and cross sections of vessels.

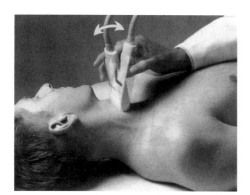

Fig. 101.1 a

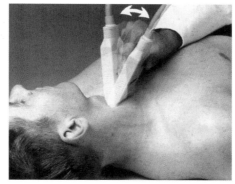

Fig. 101.1 b

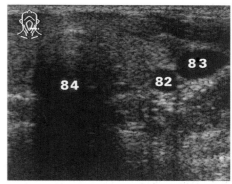

Fig. 101.1 c

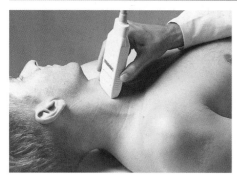

Fig. 101.2 a

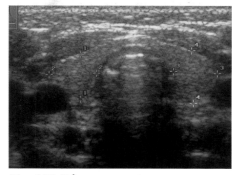

Fig. 101.2 b

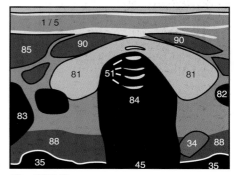

Fig. 101.2 c

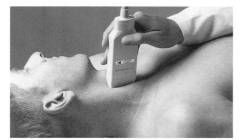

Fig. 101.3 a

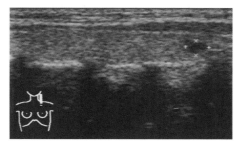

Fig. 101.3 b

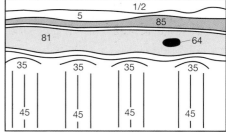

Fig. 101.3 c

Goiter

In regions where dietary intake of iodine is suboptimal, the most common diffuse thyroid disorder is iodine deficiency goiter, i.e., diffuse enlargement of the thyroid gland. Compared with their normal appearance (**Fig. 101.2**), both lobes of the thyroid are enlarged and thickened, often with a thickened isthmus as well. The iodine deficiency frequently leads to isoechoic nodules (✎) within the goiter. Where they occur peripherally, they can cause protrusion of the organ surface (**Fig. 102.3**). In chronic iodine deficiency, regressive calcifications or cysts (64 in **Fig. 102.4**) often develop in these nodules (54). With progressive degeneration, these anechoic cysts can reach a considerable size (**Fig. 102.5**) and can show central hyperechoic hemorrhages (↘ in **Fig. 102.6**).

Malignant degeneration of hyperechoic or isoechoic nodules is very rare (less than 1%). Hypoechoic thyroid nodules behave differently (see next page).

Fig. 102.1

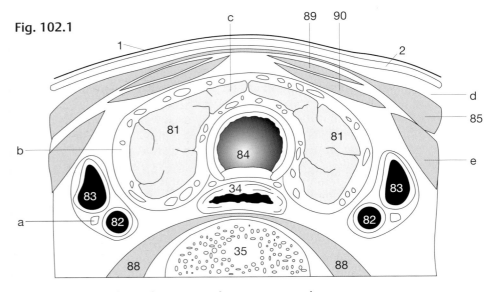

Anatomy of the thyroid region in the transverse plane

(a) Vagus nerve
(b) Fibrous capsule of thyroid
(c) Isthmus
(d) Platysma muscle
(e) Omohyoid muscle
(1) Skin
(2) Subcutaneous fatty tissue
(34) Esophagus
(35) Spine

(81) Lateral lobes of thyroid
(82) Common carotid artery
(83) Internal jugular vein
(84) Trachea
(85) Sternocleidomastoid muscle
(88) Scalenus anterior and scalenus medius muscles
(89) Sternohyoid muscle
(90) Sternothyroid muscle

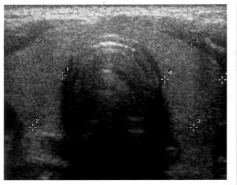

Fig. 102.2

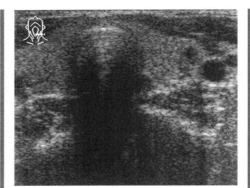

Fig. 102.4 a

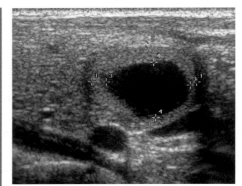

Fig. 102.5

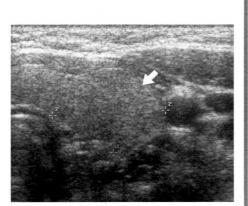

Fig. 102.3

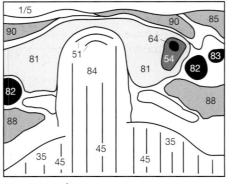

Fig. 102.4 b

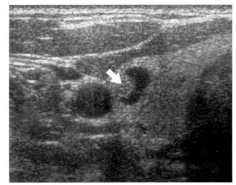

Fig. 102.6

Focal Solid Nodules

The differential diagnosis of hypoechoic thyroid lesions includes cystic degeneration and benign adenoma, but also thyroid carcinoma. Hypoechoic nodules therefore require supplementary scintigraphy.

"Hot" nodules on a scintigram are hormone-producing adenomas **(72)** and frequently appear on ultrasound scans with a hypoechoic rim within normal thyroid parenchyma **(81** in Fig. 103.1). In contrast to the typical ultrasound morphology of hepatic metastases (see p. 42), a hypoechoic rim (halo) in the thyroid gland **does not** suggest malignancy.

Nodules (54) that are **"cold" on a scintigram** and hypoechoic on ultrasound scans require further evaluation (needle aspiration for cytology or biopsy) to exclude malignancy **(Fig. 103.2)**.

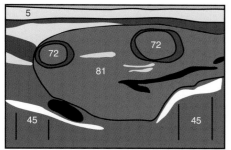

Fig. 103.1 a

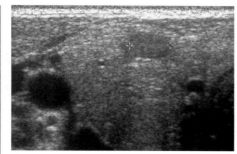

Fig. 103.2 a

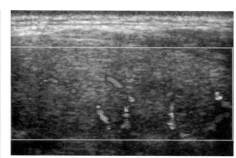

Fig. 103.3

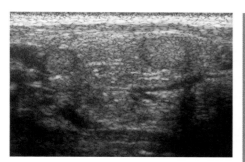

Fig. 103.1 b

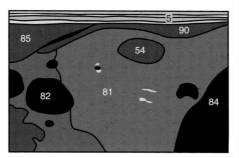

Fig. 103.2 b

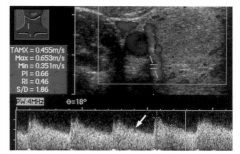

Fig. 103.4

Thyroiditis

Autoimmune Hashimoto thyroiditis leads to diffuse hypoechogenicity of the normally hyperechoic thyroid parenchyma as a result of chronic lymphocytic infiltration. In contrast to Graves disease, this hypoechogenicity persists for life. Other findings include a coarse and heterogeneous internal structure containing a proliferation of hyperperfused vessels **(Fig. 103.3)**.

Supplementary color Doppler sonography **(Fig. 103.4)** shows hyperperfusion with increased diastolic flow (✎) on the M-mode tracing (displaying blood flow as function of time). In contrast, subacute thyroiditis (de Quervain thyroiditis) is characterized by thyroid enlargement with ill-defined hypoechoic areas within zones of normal echogenicity.

Thyroid Gland – Volumetric Measurements

Unlike other European countries Germany does not iodize drinking water, and therefore must be regarded as one of the few remaining regions with suboptimal dietary intake of iodine. This must be considered when evaluating thyroid volume. Whereas statistical mean values for the German population are "normal" values, they do not reflect the normal physiologic case.

Normal Thyroid Volume

Girls younger than 15 years have a slightly higher thyroid volume than boys. To better answer the question as to whether iodine prophylaxis is indicated, the upper threshold values in milliliters are listed separately for iodine deficiency (black numbers) and for adequate iodine intake (blue numbers).

Age	Females	Males
Newborns	< 2.3 (1.5)	< 3.5 (2.0)
1 – 4 years	< 4.7 (3.0)	< 3.8 (2.9)
5 – 10 years	< 6.5 (5.0)	< 6.0 (5.4)
11 – 12 years	< 14.6 (14.1)	< 13.9 (13.2)
Adults	< 18.0	< 25.0

The blue numbers in parentheses represent the normal values for children in countries without iodine deficiency. The highest thyroid volumes accepted as normal are listed here for both lobes together, calculated according to the volume formula 0.5 x A x B x C. The mean volumes can be considerably lower.

Enlarged lymph nodes **(55)** appear as oval hypoechoic masses and are often located in vicinity of the cervical neurovascular bundle **(Fig. 104.1)** along the internal jugular vein **(83)** and carotid artery **(82)**, but also in the submental region. Physiologic lymph nodes that show reactive enlargement in the setting of viral or bacterial infection are usually elongated, with a ratio of longitudinal diameter to transverse diameter (L/T ratio) of over 2.0. They can also appear in groups **(Fig. 104.2)**. A lymph node exhibiting an L/T ratio over 2 with a central hyperechoic hilum (⬇ in **Fig. 104.3**) and a prominent hilar vascular pattern (see pp. 105, 106) can be evaluated as benign.

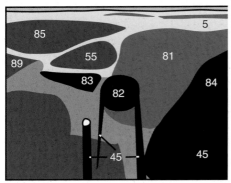

Fig. 104.1 a

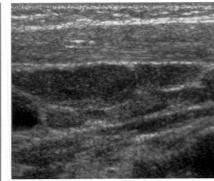

Fig. 104.2 a

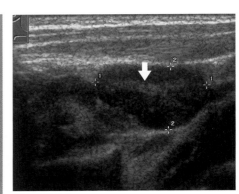

Fig. 104.3 a

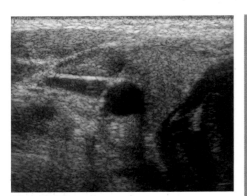

Fig. 104.1 b

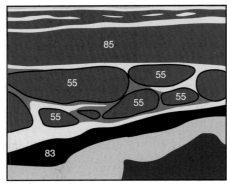

Fig. 104.2 b

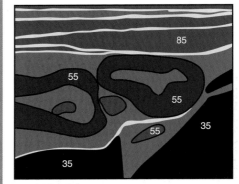

Fig. 104.3 b

In contrast, thickened, spherical lymph nodes with an L/T ratio around 1.0 without a hilum sign are suspicious for pathologic enlargement due to a process such as lymphoma or metastasis, which can occasionally show central necrosis (↖ in **Fig. 104.4**).

Infants tend to develop more severe nodal swelling than adults even in the setting of secondary inflammatory reactions. Occasionally they even develop abscesses with anechoic liquefaction in the affected lymph nodes, which can also appear as anechoic areas. Wherever such nodal abscesses are found, one must evaluate whether surgical excision and decompression are indicated.

When in doubt, additional criteria for differential diagnosis can be applied. These include visualizing the branching pattern of the intranodal blood vessels on color-coded duplex sonography, determining the pulsatility index (PI) or resistance index (RI) at that site, and quantifying tissue elasticity, "elastography". You will find examples of typical cases on the next few pages.

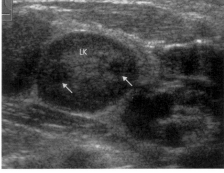

Fig. 104.4

Benign vs. Malignant Lymph Nodes

Criteria	Benign	Malignant
Ratio length / width	> 2.0	~ 1.0
Hilus sign	Positive	Negative
Vascularization	Centered in the hilus	Diffuse or branching

Differential Diagnostic Criteria

The L/T ratio described on the previous page can only be correctly calculated when you rotate the transducer 180° around the axis of its cord over the center of the lymph node. A lymph node that appears to have a low L/T ratio (**Fig. 105.1**) may then show an oval L/T ratio of 3.0 as the visualization more closely approaches its "true" diameter (**Fig. 105.2**). Although its hilar architecture is preserved (↗) there may indeed be metastatic infiltration in such an elongated lymph node (↓ in **Fig. 105.2**). Especially when higher center frequencies over 10 MHz are used, it is occasionally possible to demonstrate multiple metastases in a single lymph node (↓ ↓ in **Fig. 105.3**).

As the metastasis grows, the L/T ratio approaches the value for a sphere (1.0) (**Fig. 105.4**). However, lymphomas usually respect the capsule and tend to grow and displace tissue only within the affected lymph node (**Fig. 105.5**). In contrast, advanced metastases later infiltrate the capsule (↙ ↙) and can then spread to surrounding tissue (**Fig. 105.6**).

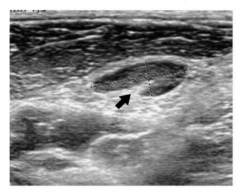

Fig. 105.1 Cross section of lymph node.

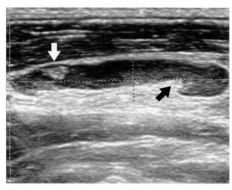

Fig. 105.2 Longitudinal section of lymph node with a small metastasis.

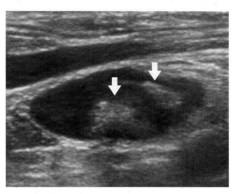

Fig. 105.3 Two lymph node metastases.

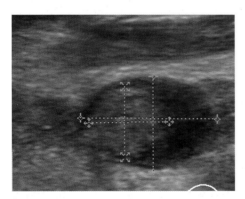

Fig. 105.4 Advanced lymph node metastasis is nearly spherical.

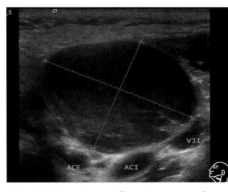

Fig. 105.5 Normally intact capsule in lymphoma.

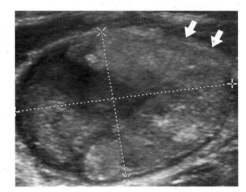

Fig. 105.6 Metastasis with capsular infiltration.

Perfusion Parameters

Where perfusing vessels can be measured within the lymph node, PI values < 1.6–1.8 and RI values < 0.8–0.9 suggest a benign process (**Fig. 105.7**), whereas PI and RI values above this gray area are more typical of malignancy (**Fig. 105.8**). However, these are not absolute threshold values but approximate values.

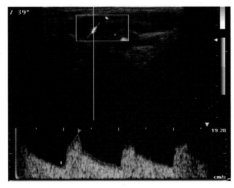

Fig. 105.7 Reactive inflammatory lymph node with PI=1.37, RI=0.73.

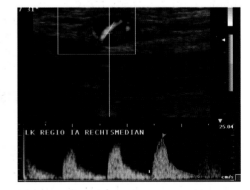

Fig. 105.8 Malignant node with PI=2.27, RI=0.92.

Differential Diagnostic Criteria

The fact that a lymph node is primarily sharply demarcated is no guarantee that it is benign. Nor does the echogenicity of a lymph node reliably identify it as malignant or benign, even though lymphomas often appear homogeneously hypoechoic (relative to adjacent muscle) and exhibit an L/T ratio of about 1 (spherical) **(Fig. 106.1)**. In contrast, the metastases of a malignant melanoma are almost invariably highly hypoechoic **(Fig. 106.2)**.

The intranodal perfusion pattern on color–coded duplex sonography is another differentiating criterion. An infiltrating lymphoma typically exhibits a treelike perfusion pattern **(Fig. 106.3)** that can often be traced into the periphery.

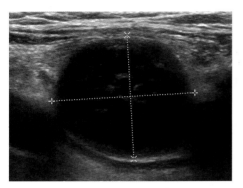

Fig. 106.1　Homogeneously hypoechoic lymphoma.

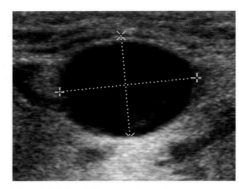

Fig. 106.2　Metastatic melanoma often highly hypoechoic.

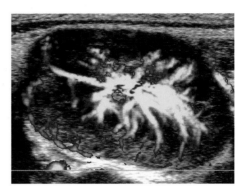

Fig. 106.3　Tree-like perfusion in lymphoma.

Reactive Inflammatory Lymph Node Enlargement

In contrast, benign lymph nodes usually exhibit intact hilar architecture (⬇ in **Fig. 106.4**) and a central pattern of perfusion that <u>cannot</u> be traced into the periphery **(Fig. 106.5)**, [7.1].

Lymph Node Metastases

Lymph node metastases, on the other hand, exhibit an irregular perfusion pattern that can be traced into the periphery of the node **(Fig. 106.6)**. Findings may also include central liquefaction **(Fig. 106.7)**.

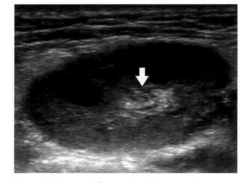

Fig. 106.4　Hilum sign in reactive inflammatory lymph node.

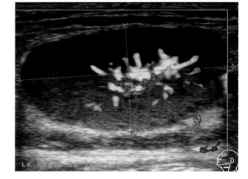

Fig. 106.5　Central perfusion in benign lymph node.

On elastography the malignant lymph nodes usually show stiffer (higher) values (here encoded in red) > 2 **(Fig. 106.8)** compared with the reactive inflammatory lymph nodes, although the accuracy of this method is still limited (depending on the examiner's experience, sensitivity is only about 62% and specificity is about 84% [7.2]).

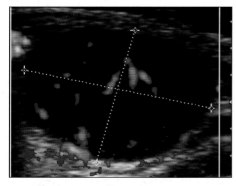

Fig. 106.6　Irregular perfusion in malignant nodal metastasis.

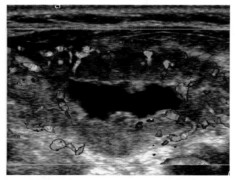

Fig. 106.7　... into the periphery occasionally with central necrosis.

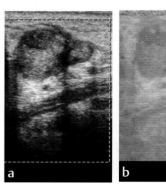

Fig. 106.8　Elastography of metastasis: values often > 2.

[7.1]　Mende U. Radiologische Bildgebung von Lymphknoten in Diagnostik und Verlaufskontrolle. Radiologie Up2date 2002; 2: 141–164

[7.2]　Bhatia CSS, Cho CCM, Yuen CYH et al. Real-time qualitative ultrasound elastography of cervical lymph nodes in routine clinical practice: Interobserver agreement and correlation with malignancy. Ultrasound in Med & Biol 2010; 36: 1990–1997

Preparation

Early exclusion of hip dysplasia in a newborn requires precision. It is also crucial to perform the various steps of the examination quickly before the newborn becomes restless. A changing table with tray is placed in the examining room or adjoining room to allow the mother or the person accompanying the child to change the diaper and clean the newborn if necessary. A heat lamp over the examination table will prevent the newborn from becoming cold **(Fig. 107.1)**.

Positioning the Newborn

The physician places the newborn in a special positioning cushion in a precise 90° lateral position. Then the mother can place her left hand beneath the newborn's head and her right hand on the upper shoulder. Most term infants exhibit strong flexion and react to unexpected extension of their legs with resistance and restlessness. Experienced examiners take care not to extend the upper leg more than necessary. The edge of the examiner's left hand gently presses the infant's thigh to prevent anteversion of the femoral neck. The goal is to obtain moderate extension in slight internal rotation **(Fig. 107.2)**, <u>without</u> allowing the knee to move forward (↓) past the edge of the positioning cushion into external rotation as shown in **Fig. 107.3**. A foot switch is used to freeze the image so that the examiner has both hands free for positioning the newborn and guiding the transducer.

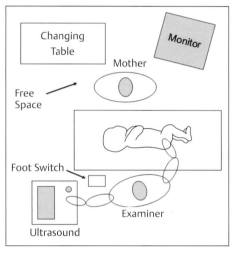

Fig. 107.1   Setting in the ultrasound suite.

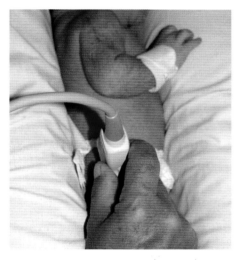

Fig. 107.2   Positioning the newborn

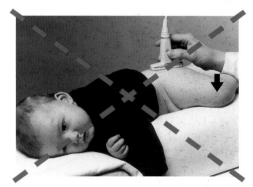

Fig. 107.3   Positioning error

Ultrasound Documentation

The German Quality Assurance Agreement on the Infant Hip requires that each hip be photographed twice and measured once at a minimum of 1.7 power magnification in the standard plane defined by Graf without any tilt. The following structures must be clearly identifiable: the osteochondral junction (line of the growth plate between the ossified femoral shaft and the cartilaginous femoral head and greater trochanter), the femoral head **(153)**, the fold of the transition from the joint capsule to the perichondrium of the femoral neck, the joint capsule itself, the acetabular labrum **(158)**, the cartilaginous acetabular roof, the ilium **(112)** including its inferior margin, and the bony promontory of the acetabular rim **(159 =** transition point, see p. 108) **(Fig. 107.5)**. Once the inferior margin of the ilium has been clearly visualized, the usability test is performed: The imaging plane is centered on the inferior margin of the ilium by rotating the transducer around the axis of the cord **(Fig. 108.6)** and corrected to obtain the median imaging plane. The acetabular labrum will then be visualized without having to search for it.

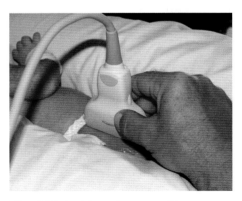

Fig. 107.4   Transducer position

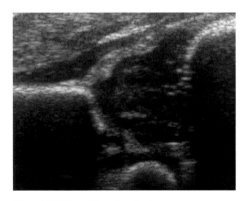

Fig. 107.5a   Standard plane

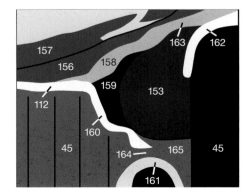

Fig. 107.5b   Anatomic diagram

P

Graf favors an image in which the ilium is visualized perpendicular to the upper margin of the image. Yet many radiologists, internists, and pediatricians prefer the orientation they are more familiar with: Here, cranial structures are visualized along the left margin of the image and the lateral structures close to the transducer appear along the upper margin of the image. However, Graf maintains that there might be evidence that this manner of visualization may be associated with a higher error rate.

First the baseline is drawn: This line originates at the "Z point" (the insertion of the rectus femoris tendon on the ilium) and extends distally, tangential and parallel to the sharply demarcated ilium with the hip extended (Fig. 108.1). Then the inferior margin of the ilium (↓ in Fig. 108.2) and the center of the lateral acetabular labrum (✭ in Fig. 108.3) are identified.
To determine the angle alpha of the bony roof, this inferior margin of the ilium (↓ in Fig. 108.2) is identified and using that as a center of rotation, a tangential line is drawn along the bony acetabulum (Fig. 108.5).

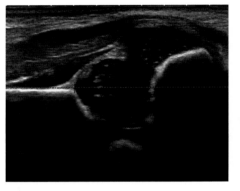

Fig. 108.1   Baseline at the ilium.

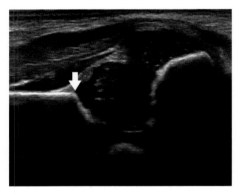

Fig. 108.2   Inferior margin of the ilium.

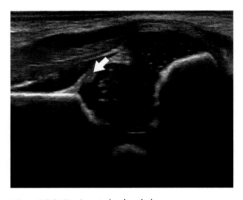

Fig. 108.3   Acetabular labrum

To construct the line for the cartilage roof angle beta (β), one first determines the transition point according to the concave–convex rule by moving laterally along the concavity of the acetabulum from the inferior margin of the ilium. After an acoustic interruption, the convex curve extends cranially along the ilium. The transition point (➚) lies at that point where the acetabular concavity joins the convexity. It can be readily identified by the acoustic interruption (Fig. 108.4).
The correct imaging plane is found by having the examiner rotate the transducer around the axis of its cord or, respectively, counterclockwise (↶ in Fig. 108.6): If he or she rotates the cranial part of the transducer too far anteriorly, the

line of the ilium will also course obliquely to the transducer as in Fig. 109.2.
The farther the acoustic shadow extends medial to the bony promontory, the more the hip is ossified. In a type I hip with an angular promontory, the transition point lies directly in the bony acetabular promontory. A line is now drawn laterally from this transition point through the center of the acetabular labrum (Fig. 108.5). The rule for identifying a type IIc unstable but still centered hip and differentiating it from a type D decentering hip (critical range hip) is as follows: The β value determines the hip type where the beta angle value is more than 77°.

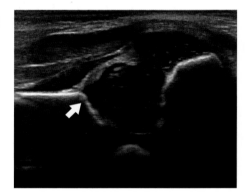
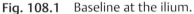

Fig. 108.4   Bony promontory

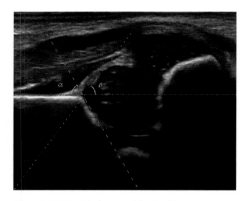

Fig. 108.5   Alpha and beta lines.

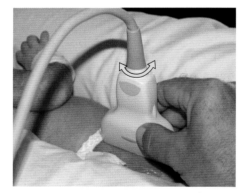

Fig. 108.6   Rotating the transducer

[7.3]   Graf R. Sonographie der Säuglingshüfte und therapeutische Konsequenzen. 6. Aufl. 2010, Thieme, Stuttgart

P

Setup and Measurement Errors

Especially in a restless newborn, it is easy for the examiner to lose the imaging plane. Where the transducer tilts posteriorly (✔ in **Fig. 109.1a**) this usually produces a medially convex, curved course (↓) of the ilium **(Fig 109.1b)** away from the transducer. However, where the transducer is tilted anteriorly **(Fig. 109.2a)** or rotated **(Fig. 108.6)**, the echo of the ilium approaches the transducer obliquely (↗ ↗ in **Fig. 109.2b**). Angling the transducer too far cranially **(Fig. 109.3a)** also visualizes the course of the ilium obliquely **(Fig. 109.3b)** and often makes it impossible to clearly visualize its inferior margin.

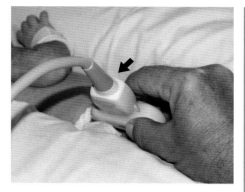

Fig. 109.1a   Posterior tilt

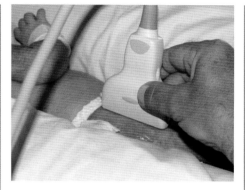

Fig. 109.2a   Anterior tilt

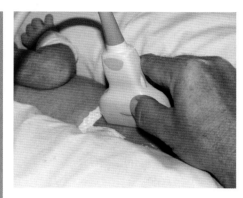

Fig. 109.3a   Cranial angulation

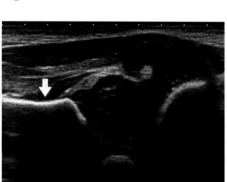

Fig. 109.1b   Posterior error plane

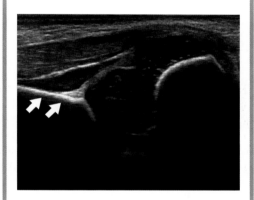

Fig. 109.2b   Anterior error plane

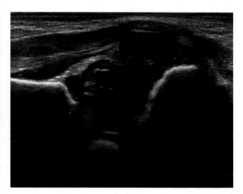

Fig. 109.3b   Cranial error plane

If the examiner angles the transducer too far caudally **(Fig. 109.4a)**, the line of the ilium also courses obliquely and the osteochondral junction is often no longer identifiable **(Fig. 109.4b)**. Because of the many sources of error and the great clinical significance of this screening examination, it is best performed by experienced examiners.

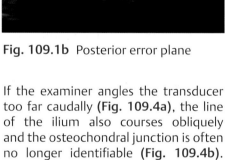

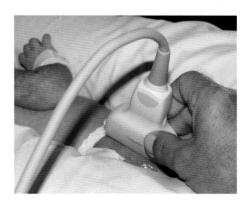

Fig. 109.4a   Caudal angulation

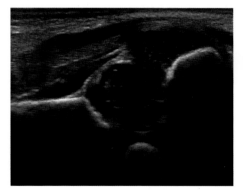

Fig. 109.4b   Caudal error plane

Classification of Infant Hips According to Graf [7.3]

In hip dysplasia, the femoral head (✳) increasingly migrates superolaterally. On the radiograph (Fig. 110.2), the bony acetabular roof is no longer close to the horizontal line (➡) but courses laterally at a steeper cranial angle (➚). The MR image (Fig. 110.3) shows the extreme case of a dislocated femoral head (✳) and an empty acetabulum (➘) that is obvious in comparison with the contralateral side. The alpha angle measured on ultrasound decreases with increasing severity of the dysplasia.

As a rule of thumb, rapid growth should cause the alpha angle to expand from a minimum postpartum angle of 50° to an angle of at least 60° by the beginning of the fourth month of life. Statistically, the optimum alpha angle is 64°. The maturation curve shows a very strong, exponential increase only in the first few weeks of life, after which it continues at a plateau. Therefore, it is important to make the diagnosis as early as possible so that adequate therapy appropriate to the

Classification of Infant Hips according to Graf	Alpha	Beta	Femoral head
I (normal)	> 60 °	< 55 °	centered
II a+	56 – 59 °	55 – 70 °	centered
II a-	50 – 55 °	55 – 70 °	centered
II g	44 – 49 °	55 – 77 °	centered
II d	44 – 49 °	> 77 °	centered
III (eccentric)	< 44 °	> 77 °	eccentric
IV (dislocated)	< 44 °	undetermined	dislocated

stage of the disorder can be promptly initiated to stabilize the femoral head and securely center it within the acetabulum. For example a type IIa- hip (Fig. 110.1) persisting after the age of 6 weeks represents defective maturation. For further detailed information, consult the extensive monograph by Reinhard Graf (see at the foot of page 108).

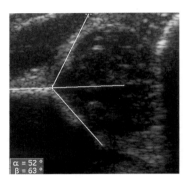

Fig. 110.1

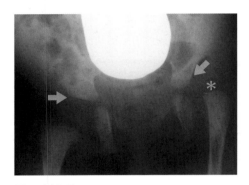

Fig. 110.2

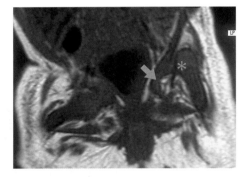

Fig. 110.3

Transient synovitis of the hip

Thickened synovia and joint effusion are typical findings of acquired hip disorders. The child is positioned supine and examined with a high-frequency linear transducer placed on the anterior hip (Fig. 110.4a). The normal joint space (168) appears as a thin anechoic space between the hyperechoic joint capsule (163) and the anterior contour of the femoral epiphysis (166) and metaphysis (167 in Fig. 110.4b). The indentation of the femoral growth plate (107) is easily identified. Measurements of the height of the epiphysis (↔) obtained on follow-up examinations can easily establish a loss of height such as can occur in necrosis of the femoral head.

A transient joint effusion frequently develops in the setting

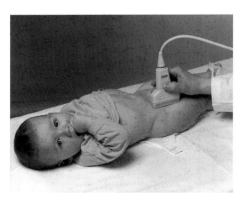

Fig. 110.4 a

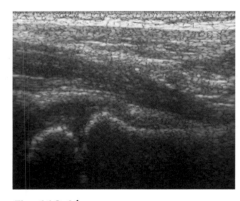

Fig. 110.4 b

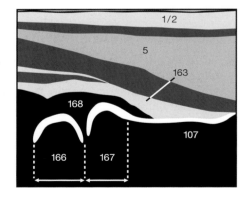

Fig. 110.4 c

of viral infection and appears as anechoic widening (⬇ ⬇) of the joint space (Fig. 110.5). A joint effusion that persists longer than two weeks or an edematous, anechoic thickening of the joint capsule suggests Legg–Calvé–Perthes disease or septic arthritis, which should be excluded by clinical and laboratory tests or supplementary MRI studies.

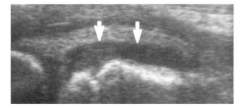

Fig. 110.5

Here are a few questions for the head and neck region. You will find the answers on the preceding pages. The answer to the image question is on page 125.

1. Topic hydrocephaly: Please list here all five normal values for the internal and subarachnoidal CSF spaces in the term newborn. What do the common acronyms for the respective measurements stand for (compound terms)?

Acronym	Compound term	Upper normal value for term newborns
SCW		< mm
CCW		< mm
IHW		< mm
LVW		< mm
3rd VW		< mm

2. Draw a sketch of the adjacent **Figure 111.1** that copies it as exactly as possible and annotate each anatomic detail you recognize on the image. Thereafter, add to the sketch where and at what angle you would have measured the external subarachnoidal CSF spaces and ventricles (see question 1). Finally, you should consider which normal variant is present in this sample image.

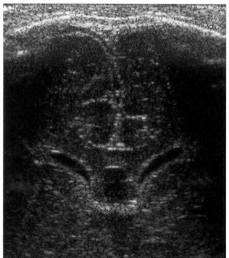

Fig. 111.1 a

Fig. 111.1 b

3. What criteria do you know for distinguishing between benign and malignant enlargement of lymph nodes? List at least 3 criteria for physiologic and malignant nodal enlargement.

Benign Criteria	Malignant Criteria

4. How do benign thyroid adenomas typically (not necessarily) appear? What criteria taken together are suspicious for thyroid malignancy?

Q

P

FAST

The **FAST** method (**F**ocused **A**ssessment with **S**onography for **T**rauma) represents a new technique for quickly and reliably excluding or confirming bleeding into the serous cavities of the chest and abdomen in trauma patients. This standardized method [7.4–7.6] is also suitable for diagnosing parenchymal tears in the spleen or liver.

Trauma patients are usually supine in the ambulance, emergency room, or shock room. Therefore, the examiner must consider where gravity will cause relevant hemorrhages to collect. From a lateral view of the torso of a supine patient **(Fig. 112.1)** it becomes apparent that free fluid will primarily collect in the pouch of Douglas in the true pelvis (🠗) and in the cranial portion of the peritoneal cavity. This pattern of distribution (anatomic predilection) is essentially attributable to the lumbar lordosis (🠕). Free fluid in the pleural cavities (in this case hemothorax) also drains posteriorly into the costodiaphragmatic recess (🠖) unless prevented from doing so by the presence of extensive pleural adhesions from previous pleuritis, which is rare.

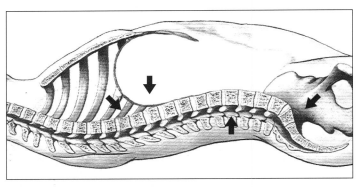

Fig. 112.1

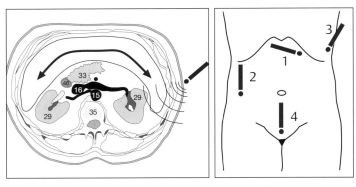

Fig. 112.2   Fig. 112.3

The hematoma is also lateralized on both sides within the abdominal cavity. This is because the spine causes anterior protrusion of the overlying median peritoneum relative to its lateral periphery **(Fig. 112.2)**. As a result, one rarely finds larger accumulations of blood close to the midline because the intraperitoneal hematoma follows gravity and drains laterally and posteriorly (⟳). Accordingly, the transducer positions shown in **Fig. 112.3** are now internationally accepted for rapid evaluation.

First the transducer is placed on the epigastrium in the transverse plane and tilted caudally **(Fig. 112.4a)** to evaluate the heart and pericardium for possible hemopericardium. Such a hemorrhage will be detectable as an anechoic rim of fluid **(79)** in the circular marginal spaces around the cardiac cavities **(115, 116** in **Fig. 112.4b)**.

The **second transducer position** on the right anterior axillary line also covers a right anechoic hemothorax **(69** in **Fig. 112.5b)** and possible bleeding **(68)** into the hepatorenal recess (pouch of Morrison) between the liver **(9)** and the kidney **(29) (Fig. 112.5c)**.

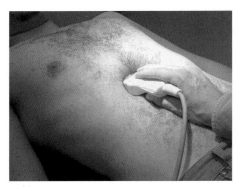

Fig. 112.4 a

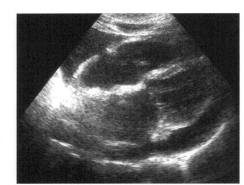

Fig. 112.4 b

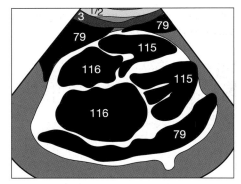

Fig. 112.4 c

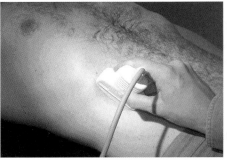

Fig. 112.5 a

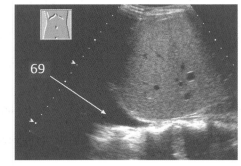

Fig. 112.5 b

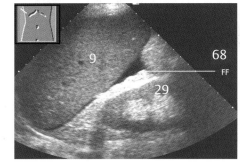

Fig. 112.5 c

The **third transducer position** on the left posterior axillary line (**Fig. 113.2a**) is used to detect not only left hemothorax (as in **Fig. 112.5b**) but also rupture of the spleen (**50** in **Fig. 113.2b**) or hemorrhage into the recess between the spleen (**37**) and left kidney (**29**) (**Fig. 113.2c**). The transducer must be angled anteriorly so that the sweep also includes the posterior costo-diaphragmatic recess and perisplenic space (**Fig. 113.1**).

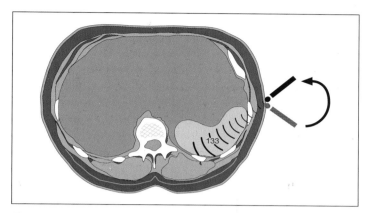

Fig. 113.1

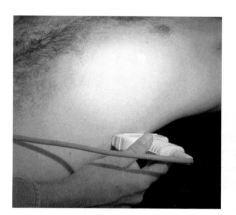

Fig. 113.2 a

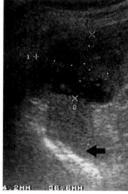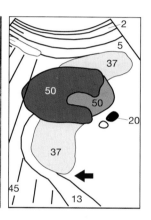

Fig. 113.2 b

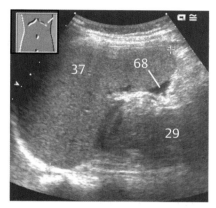

Fig. 113.2 c

Fourth transducer position: Finally, the transducer is placed on the median suprapubic region in the sagittal plane and angled caudally (**Fig. 113.3a**) to evaluate the pouch of Douglas between bowel loops (**46**), bladder (**38**), and rectum (**43**) and detect any blood (**68**) there (**Fig. 113.3b**). In larger hematomas, hemorrhage may also be detectable on the roof of the bladder and anterior to the bladder (if full).

An experienced examiner can perform the entire FAST examination without photo documentation in as little as 20–30 seconds (hence the name).

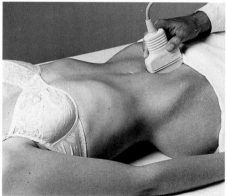

Fig. 113.3 a

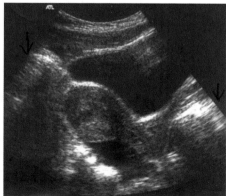

Fig. 113.3 b

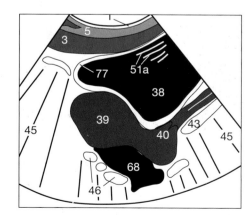

Fig. 113.3 c

[7.4] Ligawi SS, Buckley AR. Focused abdominal US in patients with trauma. Radiology. 2000 Nov; 217 (2): 426–429

[7.5] Rose JS. Ultrasound in abdominal trauma. Emerg Med Clin North AM. 2004 Aug; 22 (3): 518–599

[7.6] Brooks A, Davies B, Smethhurst M, Connolly J. Prospective evaluation of non-radiologist emergency abdominal ultrasound for haemoperitoneum. Emerg Med J. 2004 Sep; 21 (3): e5

On the pages with the quiz questions, I suggested the approach of using drawing exercises to help you memorize tomographic anatomy. How is this supposed to work?

It works with surprisingly little effort: The idea is to draw and label specific standard planes from memory (in the cafeteria on a napkin during a coffee break, or at night on any piece of paper) with long intervals in between. Do not spend more than two minutes on this exercise!

Then fill in your gaps using the diagram templates copied from this page. You just have to keep these copies with you (in your lab coat pocket). Only begin a new attempt after this exercise has left your short-term memory (> 2 – 4 hours). You will be surprised how few attempts it takes to master the tomographic anatomy if you pursue these tasks with a little determination. Have fun with it . . .

Sagittal upper abdomen, left paramedian plane (AO)

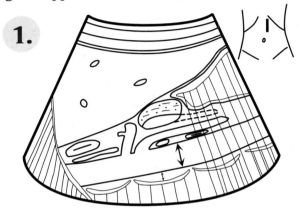

Sagittal upper abdomen, right paramedian plane (IVC)

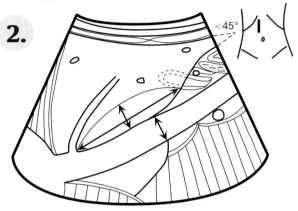

Oblique lower abdomen, para-iliac plane

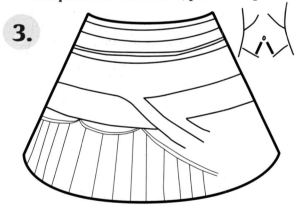

Transverse epigastric upper abdomen (celiac trunk)

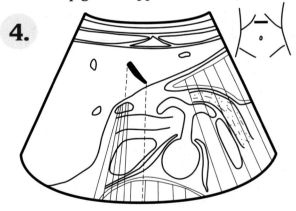

Transverse upper abdomen (renal vein crossing)

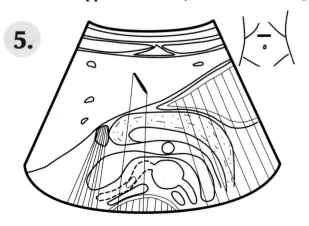

Oblique right upper abdomen (porta hepatis)

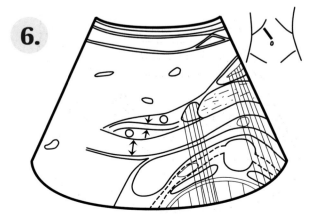

Please label the vessels and organs yourself (referring back to the previous pages where necessary) so that you can better memorize them.

These diagrams naturally represent idealized situations, and the structures they show are not always visualized in the same plane in every patient. Yet this is not important. What matters is that you know where to look for, say, the pancreas or the origins of the renal arteries in obese patients with limited sonographic visibility. Most physicians are visual learners, and you are most likely one as well.

With time, you will develop a "visual template" of the normal findings in every standard plane, and you will immediately notice any deviation ("something doesn't look right here"). That is the goal. You can even go one step further and write in the normal values where you find double-headed arrows (⟷). This will help you to memorize these values as well.

We have included a minor mistake for the advanced reader on this page. Can you find it?

Right oblique subcostal plane (hepatic venous star)

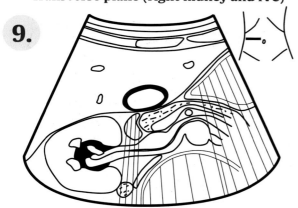

Longitudinal transhepatic plane (right kidney)

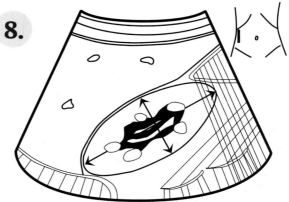

Transverse plane (right kidney and IVC)

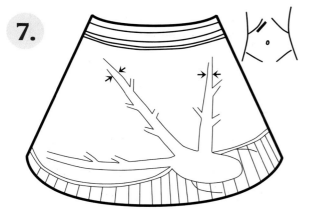

High plane of the left flank (spleen)

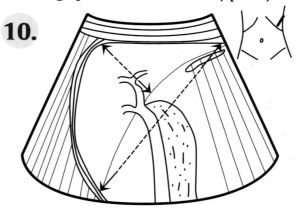

Median sagittal suprapubic plane (bladder and uterus)

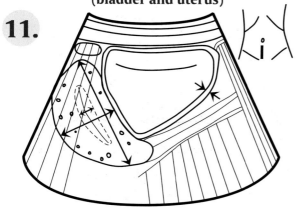

Transverse suprapubic plane (bladder and prostate gland)

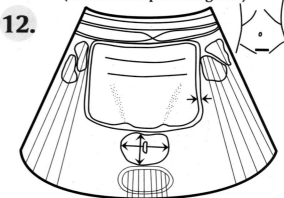

(The solutions, where to find which organ or vessel, can also be found on the internal front cover)

Primer of Ultrasound Findings

When communicating with experienced colleagues, novices are occasionally confused about which terms to use to describe findings clearly and concisely. This brief review is intended as a guide to until you have become more familiar with the common terms.

A General Description of the Sonographic Morphology of a Finding

Imaging plane?	Name the imaging plane (see front cover flap). Is the lesion visualized in the longitudinal or transverse plane?
Where?	Location, side, position within an organ or relative to other organs and vessels, i.e., central, hilar or peripheral, subcapsular, adherent to the wall.
Number?	Lesions may be focal or unifocal, multifocal, multiple, or diffusely distributed.
How large?	Specify in mm or cm. Important for follow-up examinations: Estimate progression or regression, such as can occur under therapy.
Shape?	Round, oval, spherical or stellate, wedge-shaped, geographic, irregular, thickened.
Demarcation?	Sharp (more likely benign) or ill-defined (= evidence of infiltration, as in inflammation or malignancy).
Echogenicity?	Anechoic (= homogeneous fluid), hypoechoic, or hyperechoic (possibly relative to surroundings).
Echo texture?	Homogeneous or inhomogeneous, finely granular or coarse, septated. Recently introduced categories also include elastic deformation (using special scanning technique).
Acoustic phenomena?	Acoustic shadow; edge shadow; total reflection; acoustic enhancement; section thickness, mirror image, side lobe, reverberation artifacts.
Expansion?	Displacement or infiltration of adjacent structures or vessels. Caution: mass effects can also occur with benign cysts and are therefore not necessarily a sign of malignancy.

B Useful Terms (in alphabetical order)   (⇨ application, possible meaning)

Ampullary — Developmental variant of the renal pelvis (⇨ can mimic obstruction)

Anechoic Black — (⇨ homogeneous fluids: blood, urine, bile, cyst contents, pericardial or pleural effusion)

Artifacts Illusory — Visual findings lacking physical correlates

Capsule line — Thin hyperechoic line created by the margin of an organ (⇨ absent in cirrhosis of the liver)

Comet tail — Artifact deep to pulmonary air or bowel gas

Concentric — At a pericentral location in a vessel (⇨ thrombus or calcification)

Delayed rupture — Can occur in the spleen with late hemorrhage after trauma

Density — Term is occasionally used incorrectly. The echogenicity of a tissue on an ultrasound image has little to do with its physical density

Depth compensation — Adjustment of gain to sound penetration depth

Diffuse — Distribution pattern, as in increased echogenicity

Dissection — Complication (⇨ aortic aneurysm)

Double barrel shotgun sign — Immediate adjacency of two anechoic ductal structures in the hepatic parenchyma (⇨ dilation of intrahepatic ducts parallel to portal venous branches)

Eccentric — Adherent to the wall (⇨ location of thrombus in blood vessels)

Echogenicity — "Brightness" of the pixels (increases with the number of impedance mismatches)

Ectasia — Dilation of the lumen of the abdominal aorta > 2.5–3.0 cm

Edge shadows — Acoustic phenomenon occurring deep to the edge of the gallbladder and cysts

Fluke of a whale — Typical appearance of the celiac trunk in the transverse plane

FNH — Focal nodular hyperplasia of the liver

Focal — Circumscribed lesion (focus)

Focal zone Part of the image with the highest vertical resolution

Forced inspiration Respiratory maneuver (⇨ vena cava collapse test)

Gain Amplification of received echoes when generating image

Halo Hypoechoic rim of a lesion (⇨ typical of hepatic metastases)

Haustration Convex pouching (typical of colon)

Hilum fat sign Benignity criterion for lymph nodes

Hyperechoic Bright (⇨ as in fatty degeneration of parenchymal organs)

Hypoechoic Dark, few echoes (⇨ muscle, subcutaneous fat, parenchyma)

Ill-defined Demarcation (⇨ criterion of infiltration in malignancy and inflammation)

Impedance mismatch
Interface between tissue layers with differing velocity of sound propagation that produces echoes

Infiltration Spread into adjacent structures (⇨ malignancy criterion)

Inhomogeneous Irregular pattern of distribution of echogenicity

Iris sign Typical progression of enhancement in a liver hemangioma on spiral CT

Jet sign Inflow from the ureter into the bladder on color coded Doppler studies (⇨ intrastenotic and poststenotic acceleration of flow)

Kinking Tortuous, angular course (⇨ aortic aneurysm)

L/T ratio Longitudinal diameter divided by transverse diameter (⇨ malignancy status of lymph node)

Liquefaction Usually anechoic (⇨ as in the center of abscesses, metastases)

LN Lymph node

Lobe of sound beam
The acoustic wave front has a finite thickness (⇨ section thickness artifact)

Multifocal Having several foci in a single organ

Narrowing of renal parenchyma
(⇨ Typical finding in renal degeneration)

Necrosis Hypoechoic, usually central area of liquefaction (⇨ abscess or metastasis)

Nodular Multifocal distribution pattern of lesions

Nutcracker Compression of the left renal vein by the aorta and superior mesenteric artery

Oscillating peristalsis
Back and forth motion of bowel contents

Pennate Exhibiting parallel stripes (⇨ pattern typical of muscles such as the psoas major)

Perifocal Marginal zone around a lesion

Plaque Hyperechoic calcified zone in blood vessels

Polycyclic Knobbly or resembling cauliflower (⇨ structure of tumor in the stomach or bladder)

PP index Parenchyma to pelvis index (⇨ kidney findings)

Predilection Common location of a lesion or abnormality

Pruned tree Abrupt changes in caliber of the portal vein branches (⇨ cirrhosis of the liver)

Pseudocysts (⇨ Complication of pancreatitis)

Pulsation Simple (⇨ arteries such as aorta), double (⇨ veins such as inferior vena cava)

Rarefaction Decreased vascularity (⇨ cirrhosis of the liver)

Respecting Failure to invade vascular structures is inconsistent with infiltrative growth (⇨ benignity criterion)

Reverberation Repetitive echoes (artifact)

Section thickness artifact
Apparently ill-defined border of an obliquely sectioned hollow organ (⇨ important to consider in differential diagnosis of gallbladder sludge or bladder sediment)

Septate, septated
Anechoic hollow spaces are divided by hyperechoic lines (⇨ cysts, cystic ovarian tumors; ⇨ aortic dissection)

Sharp Demarcation (⇨ benignity criterion)

Side lobe artifact
(⇨ Occurs in anechoic structures next to strong reflectors)

Sludge Hyperechoic sediment in the gallbladder

Spoke-wheel pattern
Pattern of echogenicity (⇨ focal nodular hyperplasia of the liver, ⇨ septation in echinococcal cysts)

Starry sky Multiple hyperechoic focal lesions (⇨ in tuberculosis of the spleen)

Stenosis Narrowing of a vessel or hollow organ

Stent Tube implanted to maintain patency of vascular or ductal stenosis

String of pearls Configuration of the medullary pyramids along the border between the parenchyma and renal pelvis (⇨ pattern of dilation of the pancreatic duct in pancreatitis)

Target sign Concentric circles of alternating echogenicity (⇨ intussusception; differential diagnosis: bowel wall inflammation)

Thickening Variation in shape (⇨ margins of the liver in hepatic disorders)

Total reflection A black shadow occurs deep to bone and air

Trackball Control device on the ultrasound unit

Triangular Typical three-sided configuration (⇨ organ infarcts)

Vena cava collapse test
Examination maneuver using forced inspiration (⇨ in suspected right heart failure)

Wall thickness Diagnostic criterion (⇨ hollow organs, vascular structures)

Wedge-shaped Pattern of increased parenchymal echogenicity (⇨ typical pattern in infarct)

The following list contains terms that are applicable to certain organ systems. For each organ, terms for spatial orientation are listed, followed by typical ultrasound changes that may provide information about the underlying disorder. Then any features and considerations specific to the organ are listed. This section is intended as a concise, time-saving review.

Liver
Spatial terms
- Subdiaphragmatic, subcapsular ⟷ perihilar, central; specify segment (not only lobe), periportal, parahepatic, focal ⟷ diffuse

Typical morphology
⇨ Possible diagnosis
- Diffuse increase in echogenicity ⇨ Fatty liver
- Diffuse loss of sound penetration with depth ⇨ Fatty liver
- Geographic, sharply demarcated differences in echogenicity around the gallbladder bed or near the portal bifurcation ⇨ Focal fatty infiltration or focal sparing in fatty infiltration
- Spherical anechoic and sharply demarcated lesions with edge shadows and distal acoustic enhancement ⇨ Benign cysts
- Septated cysts ⇨ Echinococcosis (spleen involved?)
- Singular or multiple lesions with hypoechoic rim (= halo) ⇨ Metastases
- Spherical hyperechoic and sharply demarcated lesion without halo ⇨ Hemangioma
- Double barrel shotgun sign along portal vein branches ⇨ Dilated intrahepatic bile ducts
- Intraductal hyperechoic, oval lesions with acoustic shadowing ⇨ Gallstones or air in the bile ducts
- Absent capsule line, peripherally rarefied vessels, thickened organ edges and "pruned portal tree" ⇨ Cirrhosis (shrunken liver only in late-stage disease)

Specific considerations
- Differential diagnosis may require contrast harmonic imaging and elastographic techniques
- Spiral CT: Dynamic study with typical contrast enhancement pattern diagnostic of hemangioma: "iris sign"

Gallbladder
Spatial terms
- Endoluminal, adherent to the wall, infundibular, fundal

Typical morphology
⇨ Possible diagnosis
- Hypoechoic, multilayered, edematous wall thickening, possibly with perifocal ascites ⇨ Acute cholecystitis
- Hyperechoic intraluminal sedimentation ⇨ Sludge (differential diagnosis: section thickness, reverberation, and side lobe artifacts)
- Hyperechoic, spherical–to–oval intraluminal lesion with distal acoustic shadowing ⇨ Cholecystolithiasis
- Focal wall thickening or hyperechoic lesion adherent to the wall without acoustic shadow ⇨ Polyp

Spleen
Spatial terms
- Subdiaphragmatic, subcapsular ⟷ central, perihilar, perisplenic, parasplenic

Typical morphology
⇨ Possible diagnosis
- Thickened organ shape ⇨ Splenomegaly in viral infection, lymphoma or portal hypertension
- Triangular or wedge-shaped area of decreased echogenicity ⇨ Suggests infarct, ⇨ color Doppler
- Inhomogeneous patchy parenchyma ⇨ Suggests lymphomatous infiltration
- Parasplenic round mass isoechoic to spleen ⇨ Accessory spleen, lymph node
- Hypoechoic, bandlike discontinuity in the parenchyma, possibly with subcapsular hypoechoic fluid ⇨ Suggests splenic rupture (free abdominal fluid?)

Pancreas
Spatial terms
- Head, uncinate process, body, tail, disseminated, peripancreatic, lesser sac

Typical morphology
⇨ Possible diagnosis
- Diffuse increase in echogenicity ⇨ Lipomatosis
- Hypoechoic edematous enlargement, applying pressure to transducer is painful, anechoic peripancreatic fluid may be present ⇨ Acute pancreatitis
- Organ atrophy with focal hyperechoic calcifications with acoustic shadowing, possibly with irregular dilation of the pancreatic duct ⇨ Chronic pancreatitis
- Anechoic, cystic cavity in the pancreatic region ⇨ Pseudocyst (differential diagnosis: fluid-filled bowel loop)

Specific considerations
- Endoscopic ultrasound allows intraluminal visualisation through the stomach

Adrenal Glands
Typical morphology
⇨ Possible diagnosis
- Unilateral or bilateral hypoechoic thickening ⇨ Adenoma (differential diagnosis: metastasis)

Specific considerations
- Differential diagnostic modalities include dynamic densitometry using spiral CT (contrast washout curve)

Kidneys
Spatial terms
- Parapelvic, pelvic, perihilar ⟷ subcapsular, parenchymal, cortical, pericapsular, polar, perirenal, at the pelvic–parenchymal junction, unilateral, bilateral; do not forget to specify the side (body markers)

Typical morphology
⇨ Possible diagnosis
- Homogeneous, anechoic, round–to–oval, sharply demarcated lesion with distal acoustic enhancement ⇨ Cyst
- Homogenous, hyperechoic, sharply demarcated, spherical lesion ⇨ Angiolipoma
- Row of round hypoechoic apparent lesions without distal acoustic enhancement along the border between the parenchyma and renal pelvis resembling a string of pearls ⇨ Physiologic medullary pyramids
- Hypoechoic pelvic thickening or prominent pelvis ⇨ Urinary obstruction (differential diagnosis: pelvic cyst, ampullary renal pelvis)
- Parenchymal thinning with PP index < normal and kidney size < 10 cm ⇨ Renal atrophy
- Inhomogeneous mass with expansion ⇨ Suggests malignancy
- Hyperechoic, wedge-shaped area in the parenchyma ⇨ Suggests infarct

Specific considerations
- Differential diagnostic modalities include densitometry on spiral CT and perfusion pattern on color-coded Doppler sonography
- Ectopic kidney, horseshoe kidney
- Accessory renal arteries

Gastrointestinal Tract

Spatial terms
- Intraluminal, adherent to the wall; also specify abdominal quadrant for bowel

Typical morphology
⇨ Possible diagnosis
- Target sign (concentric structure of alternating echogenicity) ⇨ Intussusception
- Focal hypoechoic wall thickening with discontinuity of the layers of the wall ⇨ Suggests malignancy (differential diagnosis: lymphoma, more likely disseminated than focal)

Specific considerations
- Hypotonic visualization of the gastric wall is possible using water as an anechoic intraluminal medium
- Endoscopic ultrasound (of gastric and rectal wall) is an option
- Peristalsis can be provoked by rapidly alternating pressure on the transducer

Bladder

Spatial terms
- Intraluminal, adherent to the wall, intravesical, extravesical, perivesical, bladder floor, bladder roof

Typical morphology
⇨ Possible diagnosis
- Hyperechoic material with gravitational sedimentation pattern ⇨ Sludge, hematoma
- Diffuse, hypoechoic wall thickening ⇨ Cystitis
- Focal wall thickening, possibly extending into lumen as polypoid projection ⇨ Suggests malignancy
- Spherical, anechoic, sharply demarcated perivesical structure ⇨ Bladder diverticulum
- Hyperechoic intraluminal circle ⇨ Balloon of indwelling catheter (rare differential diagnosis: ureterocele in children)
- Suddenly appearing linear intraluminal inhomogeneity ⇨ Jet sign representing urine propelled from the ureteral ostium by ureteral peristalsis

Specific considerations
- Remember to clamp an indwelling catheter prior to examination so the bladder will be full and allow adequate evaluation of the bladder wall

Vessels and Retroperitoneum

Spatial terms
- Para-aortic, retro-aortic, pre-aortic, paracaval, retrocaval, precaval, aortocaval, prevertebral, retrocrural, mesenteric, para-iliac, inguinal, cervical

Typical morphology
⇨ Possible diagnosis
- Endoluminal material of varying echogenicity ⇨ Thrombus
- Diameter of thrombosed vein more than twice of that of the accompanying artery ⇨ Sign of acute thrombosis (< 10 days)
- Dilated aortic lumen containing a hyperechoic membrane ⇨ Dissected aortic aneurysm
- Hypoechoic oval structure adjacent to a vessel ⇨ Typical lymph node
- Oval lymph node (L/T ratio > 2) with hilum fat sign ⇨ Benignity criterion for lymph nodes
- Homogeneously hypoechoic spherical lymph node (L/T ratio ~ 1) without hilum fat sign ⇨ Typical of lymphoma (determine perfusion pattern on color-coded Doppler sonography)

Specific considerations
- Color-coded Doppler sonography often provides additional information

Thyroid Gland

Spatial terms
- Isthmus, lobes (specify side), subcapsular, at upper or lower pole

Typical morphology
⇨ Possible diagnosis
- Isoechoic nodular lesions with hypoechoic rim ⇨ Typical of adenoma
- Cystic anechoic lesions, often multifocal ⇨ Nodular transformation induced by iodine deficiency
- Hypoechoic nodular lesions ⇨ Suggest malignancy if scintigram shows cold lesions
- Normally hyperechoic parenchyma appears diffusely hypoechoic ⇨ Hashimoto thyroiditis
- Thyroid enlargement with ill-defined hypoechoic areas within otherwise normal echogenicity ⇨ Subacute de Quervain thyroiditis

Specific considerations
- Findings are often best interpreted together with scintigraphy and color-coded Doppler sonography

C Checklists

The third part of this review comprises the checklists, which are not repeated here to save space. They are listed on the pocket-size cards or on the following pages:

Topic	Page
Aortic aneurysm	23
Right heart failure	25
Normal values of porta hepatis	32
Portal hypertension	33
Criteria for cysts	39
Criteria for cirrhosis	41
Normal renal values, PP index	47
Width of renal pelvis in neonates	54
Grading of vesicoureteral reflux in children	55
Normal values of appendix	69
Hydrops fetalis	88
CSF spaces in neonates	95
Cerebral hemorrhage	98
Benign vs. malignant lymph nodes	104
Classification of hips according to Graf	110

3D 10, 13, 19

A
Abdominal circumference 85
Abrupt change in caliber 41
Absence of amniotic fluid 90
Accessory spleen 72
Achondroplasia 91
Acoustic enhancement 16, 37
Acoustic shadow 17
AcuNav 15
Acute transient synovitis of
   the hip 107
Adamkiewicz 23
Agenesis of the corpus
   callosum 97
Anatomy 27, 102
Aneurysm 23, 25
Angiomyolipoma 57
Aorta 21–23
Appendicitis 69
Artifacts 16–18, 67
Ascites 10, 45, 88

B
Banana sign 86
Bandwidth 7, 11
Bile ducts 32
Biliary air 40
Blood clots 60, 61
Breathing instructions 20

C
Caroli syndrome 39
Carotid plaque 15
Catheter 60, 99
Cavum of the septum
   pellucidum 97
Center frequency 7
Cerebellum 86
Cerebral atrophy 95, 97, 99
Cerebral hemorrhage 98
Cervix 77
Cholecystitis 45
Cholestasis 40, 43
Chorionic cavity 82, 84
Choroid plexus 86, 94
Cine loop 8
Cirrhosis criteria 41
Cirrhosis of the liver 41
Cleft lip and palate 88
Club foot 91
Colitis 70
Collapse test (inferior vena
   cava) 25, 36
Columns of Bertin 48
Common bile duct 32
Compound imaging 13
Concretion 44, 56, 60
Congenital cardiac shunts 89
Congested liver 35
Conn syndrome 57
Contrast agent 12, 40
Contrast enema 68
Contrast harmonic 12

Costophrenic angle 35
Crown–rump length 84
Cruveilhier–Baumgarten
   syndrome 33
CSF shunt 99
CSF spaces 94
Curtain trick (spleen) 71
Cystitis 60, 61
Cysts 39, 48, 73, 80, 81, 86, 96,
   101, 102

D
De Quervain thyroiditis 103
Delayed splenic rupture 73
Density 7
Dermoid cyst 81
Detail resolution 10
Diarrhea 69
Dilation 23, 55
Dissection 23
Diverticulitis 70
Double barrel shotgun sign 43
Double bubble sign 90
Drainage catheter 40, 69
Dromedary hump 48
Duodenal atresia 90
Duodenum 28

E
Echinococcus 39, 73
Echo 6
Echogenicity 7
Ectasia 23
Ectopic pregnancy 82
Edge shadows 17, 44
Embankment 35, 38
Endometriosis 81
Endometrium 78
Endoscopic ultrasound 30, 77
Epididymitis 76
ERCP 40, 43, 44

F
FAST 112
Fatty infiltration (liver) 38
Fatty liver 7, 37, 38
Fecal impaction 70
Femur length 85
Five-chamber view 89
Focal nodular hyperplasia 40
Follicle 80
Foramen of Monro 94
Four-chamber view 89
Freeze 8
Frequencies 6, 9

G
Gain 8
Gallbladder 35
Gallstones 44
Gel quantity 20
Gender determination 83
Goiter 102
Graafian follicle 80
Graves disease 103

H
Halo sign 42, 103
Harmonic imaging 11
Hashimoto 103
Heart defect 89
Hemangioma 39, 73
Hematometra 79
Hepatic steatosis 37
Hepatic veins 36, 38
Hepatitis 41
Hernia 67, 76
Hilum sign, hilum fat sign 24
Hip dysplasia 107–110
Hirschsprung 69
Hodgkin 24
Hydrocele 76
Hydrocephalus 86, 95, 99
Hydrops fetalis 88

I
Iliac vessels 22, 25
Image generation 6
Impedance 6
Indwelling catheter 60
Inferior vena cava 21, 22, 25, 36
Infertility 80
Intrauterine device 78
Intussusception 68
Iodine deficiency 102
Iris sign 40
IUD 78

K
Kidney failure 48

L
L/T ratio 24, 105
Legg–Calvé–Perthes
   disease 110
Lemon sign 86
Lesser sac 28
Leukemia 31, 72
Levovist 12
Light adaptation 10
Liver 35–46
Liver hemangioma 39, 40
Lymph nodes 21, 24, 31, 33,
   72, 104–106
Lymphocele 63
Lymphoma 31

M
Medullary pyramids 66
Megahertz 7, 9
Metastases 42, 57, 58
Mirror image artifact 17, 37
Missed abortion 88
Myoma 79

N
Near-field resolution 9
Nephritis 51
Nephroblastoma 58
Nephrocalcinosis 50
Nephrolithiasis 56

Neurinomas 57
Newborns 49, 58, 95
Non-Hodgkin
   lymphoma 24, 73
Nuchal translucency 88

O
Oligohydramnios 90
Omphalocele 90
Operation 8
Optison 12
Orchitis 76
Orientation 19, 27
Ormond 52
Ovulation 80

P
Pancreas 28–30
Pancreatic carcinoma 30
Pancreatitis 29,
Panorama image 10, 13
Parasites 39
Penetration depth 8, 9
Pericardial effusion 88
Peristalsis 24
Peritoneal carcinosis 30
Phase inversion technique 11
Piezoelectric effect 7
Placenta position 83
Plaque 13
Pleural effusion 10
Plexus cysts 96
Polydactyly 91
Polyps 44
Porta hepatis 32
Portal hypertension 32
Portal vein 32, 38
Position of lumen 23
Post-void residual bladder
   volume 59
Pouch of Douglas 60, 80
Pouch of Morrison 45
Precision up-sampling 14
Pregnancy testing 82
Pressure 19
Prostate carcinoma 74
Pulse compression 14
Pyloric hypertrophy 65

R
Rarefaction 41
Reflux 54, 55, 66
Rejection reaction 63
Renal atrophy 51
Renal calculi 56
Renal carcinoma 57
Renal cyst 48
Renal duplication 48, 49
Renal infarct 51, 56
Renal transplant 62, 63
Retroperitoneum 21, 24
Reverberation 16
Reverberation artifact 16, 67
Right heart failure 25, 36
Risk of rupture 23, 73

S
Section thickness artifact 16, 60
Shrunken liver 41
Side lobe 18, 60
Side lobe artifact 18
SieScape 10
Sludge 43
SonoCT 13
Sonovue 12
Sound waves 6
Spatial orientation 19, 27, 30, 77, 122
Spina bifida 87
Splenic infarct 72, 73
Splenic rupture 73
Splenomegaly 72
Starry sky (spleen) 73
Syndactyly 91

T
Target sign 67, 68
Testis 75
Tethered cord syndrome 100
Thyroid carcinoma 103
Total reflection 6
Trabeculated bladder 60
Trackball 8
Transducer pressure 19
Transducer types 9

U
Umbilical hernia 90
Undescended testis 76
Upper GI series 66
Urachus 61
Ureter dilation 55
Ureterocele 60, 61
Urinary obstruction 52, 63
Uterine carcinoma 79

V
Varicocele 76
Venous star (liver) 36
Voiding cystourethrogram 54
Volume formula 59

Y
Yolk sac 84

The currently applicable Ultrasound Agreements pursuant to § 135, paragraph 2, of the German Social Security Code, Vol. V, as amended on 6 October 1996 specify the technical requirements for equipment and the required qualifications for the examiner. However, policies regarding the type and scope of imaging documentation had not yet progressed beyond the draft stage at the time of publication of this work. Therefore, the following text can only serve as an example:

Template for report of normal findings for patient _____
Date of birth _____

The examination was performed without/with contrast agents with a _____ MHz transducer/with the following additional technology: THI / CHI / SonoCT _____.

Retroperitoneum:
The retroperitoneum is well visualized without evidence of lymph node enlargement or other pathologic masses. Aorta and inferior vena cava are unremarkable.

Pancreas:
The parenchyma is homogeneous without evidence of focal lesions or inflammation. The size of the pancreas is within the normal range / enlarged, with the head measuring _____ cm, the body _____ cm, and the tail _____ cm. The pancreatic duct is normal/ cannot be visualized / and measures _____ mm in diameter. *(Delete inapplicable text.)*

Liver:
The liver is of normal size and shape and exhibits a smooth surface. The parenchyma is homogeneous without evidence of focal masses. Echogenicity is normal. Intrahepatic biliary ducts and vessels appear normal.

Gallbladder and Bile Ducts:
The gallbladder is of normal size and ductal diameter without evidence of inflammatory wall thickening, stones, or sludge. The common bile duct is completely visualized / visualized as far as _____.

Adrenal Glands:
The beds of both adrenal glands are unremarkable without evidence of a mass.

Kidneys:
Both kidneys are well visualized, show normal respiratory mobility, and are of normal size, with the right kidney measuring _____ cm and the left kidney _____ cm in length. The parenchyma is homogeneous and of normal width in both kidneys. The PP index of the right kidney is 1:_____ and of the left kidney 1:_____. No evidence of calculi, congestion, or pathologic masses.

Spleen:
The spleen is normal in size for the patient's age, measuring _____ cm in length and _____ cm in width, and exhibits a homogeneous parenchyma. No evidence of focal lesions on the plain ultrasound scan / application of _____ reveals_____.

Abdominal Cavity:
No evidence of free fluid.

Gastrointestinal Tract:
The thickness of the gastric wall is within the normal range, measuring _____ mm. No evidence of focal thickening of the wall of the stomach, small bowel, or colon. Normal peristalsis was observed.

Bladder:
The wall has a smooth contour and normal thickness, measuring _____ mm. Normal post-void residual bladder volume of _____ mL. No evidence of calculi, diverticula, or ureterocele.

Reproductive Organs:
The **uterus** is of normal size for the patient's age, measuring _____ x _____ cm. The thickness of the endometrium multiplied by 2 is _____ mm. No evidence of retained secretion or focal masses. No evidence of free fluid in the pouch of Douglas. The ovaries are well visualized / not visualized on the (right / left) and are of normal size; the right ovary measures _____ x _____ cm and the left ovary _____ x _____ cm.
The **prostate gland** is homogeneous and of normal size, measuring _____ x _____ x _____ cm. No evidence of focal masses or calcifications. The seminal vesicles are unremarkable.

Conclusion:
Unremarkable normal findings in the abdomen and retroperitoneum. (Don't forget to address the clinical line of inquiry. *Delete inapplicable text.*)

Remarks:_____

Answer to Fig. 18.4:
The image shows a longitudinal section of the aorta (15). Its wall contains hyper-echoic calcifications (arteriosclerotic plaques, 49), with posterior acoustic shadows (45). The larger plaque could have been easily overlooked without the acoustic shadow because it is located immediately adjacent to hyperechoic (= bright) bowel gas (46), which also creates an acoustic shadow. Below (= posterior to) the aorta (15) we also see the phenomenon of distal acoustic enhancement (70).

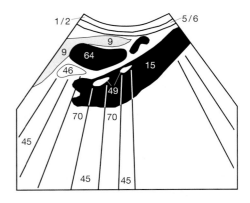

Fig. 122.1

Answer to Fig. 19.1:
Prior to beginning the practical sessions, you should become familiar with spatial orientation in a three-dimensional space. To make the first step easy, we will initially consider only two planes perpendicular to each other: the vertical (sagittal) plane (Fig. 122.2) and the horizontal (transverse) plane (Fig. 122.3).

On page 19 you were asked to use a coffee filter to help picture how the sound waves propagate through the body when the transducer is placed on the anterior abdominal wall. Both planes display the anterior abdominal wall at the upper edge of the image (up = anterior). As the convention is to view all sagittal images from the patient's right side (Fig. 122.2a), the patient's cranial structures are displayed at the left edge of the image (left = cranial) and the caudal structures at the right edge.

Rotate the transducer 90° counter-clockwise to place it in the transverse plane. As this plane is viewed from below (caudal) all the structures are reversed (left = right, Fig. 122.3b). The same imaging convention is used for transverse planes in CT and MRI. It all makes good sense: If you stand at the foot of the bed before a supine patient, the patient's liver (on the patient's right side) will be on the left in your field of view. Only neurosurgeons prefer to view cranial CT images from above as this corresponds to their intraoperative perspective.

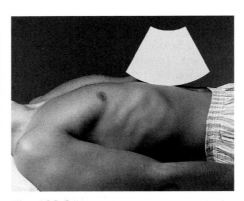

Fig. 122.2 a

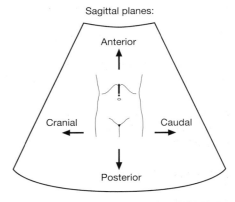

Fig. 122.2 b

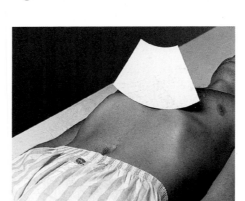

Fig. 122.3 a

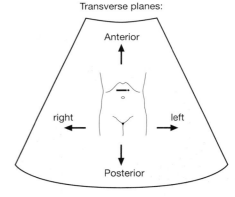

Fig. 122.3 b

Answers to Figs. 20.4–20.6:
When viewing these three images, it is apparent on the left image that the structures on the whole are more poorly visualized than usual. The image in **Fig. 20.4** seems blurred and is diffusely obscured by scatter. This is due to the typical beginner's error of applying insufficient pressure to the trans-ducer, not too little gel.

If the amount of gel is indeed inadequate or the examiner breaks the skin coupling by tilting the transducer, an image like that shown in **Fig. 20.5** will result: A black band appears along the margin of the lost coupling (here on the right side of the image) beginning immediately at the skin-transducer interface and not only in a deeper plane. This finding distin-guishes lost skin coupling from acoustic shadows behind ribs, bowel gas, gallstones, and renal calculi. In **Fig. 20.6** the same plane in the same patient was imaged a few seconds later with better coupling and sufficient pressure on the transducer. All structures are visualized far more clearly.

Answer to Fig. 26.2 (Question 7):

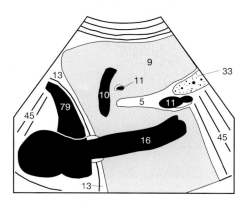

Imaging plane:
Sagittal upper abdomen, paramedian plane over the inferior vena cava **(16)**.
Organs:
Liver **(9)**, heart, and pancreas **(33)**
Structures:
Diaphragm **(13)**, hepatic vein **(10)**, portal branch **(11)**, caudate lobe **(9a)**
Significant finding:
Anechoic space **(79)** between myocardium/epicardium and diaphragm
Diagnosis:
Pericardial effusion **(79)**
Differential diagnosis:
Epicardial fat

Answer to Fig. 34.1 (Question 4):

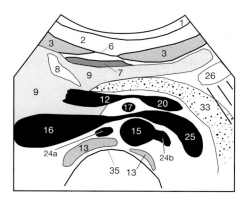

Imaging plane:
Transverse upper abdomen at the level of the renal vein crossing
Organs:
Liver **(9)**, stomach **(26)**, pancreas **(33)**
Vessels: Aorta **(15)**, inferior vena cava **(16)**, renal artery **(24)**, renal vein **(25)**, superior mesenteric artery **(17)**, confluence **(12)**
Structures:
Ligaments **(7,8)**, rectus abdominis muscle **(3)**, lumbar vertebra **(35)**
Significant finding:
Prominent lumen of the renal vein **(25)**
Diagnosis:
Still physiologic, no pathologic dilation of the left renal vein (due to nutcracker syndrome between **15** and **17**)

Answer to Fig. 46.1 (Question 5):

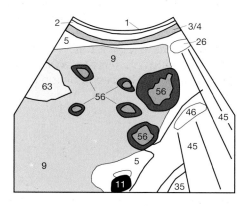

Imaging plane:
Right oblique subcostal plane
Organs:
Liver **(9)**, stomach **(26)**, small bowel **(46)**
Significant finding:
Homogeneous, hyperechoic, sharply demarcated area **(63)**, multiple round to oval intrahepatic lesions with hypoechoic rim
Diagnosis:
Focal fatty infiltration **(63)** and multiple hepatic metastases **(56)** with at least two episodes of metastatic spreading as new and older metastases are visible next to each other

Answer to Fig. 46.2 (Question 5):

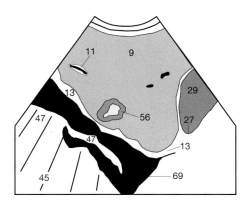

Imaging plane: Sagittal plane along the right midclavicular line
Organs:
Liver **(9)**, kidney **(29)**, lung **(47)**
Diagnosis: Subdiaphragmatic hepatic metastasis **(56)** with hypoechoic rim and pleural effusion **(69)**
Differential diagnosis: Hyperechoic appearance suggests hemangioma, but halo is inconsistent with this

Answer to Fig. 46.3 (Question 5):

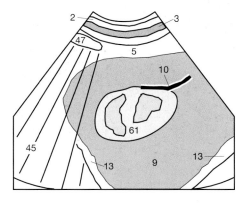

Imaging plane: Sagittal upper abdomen, right paramedian plane
Organs:
Liver **(9)**, lung **(47)**, diaphragm **(13)**
Significant finding:
Hyperechoic, partially inhomogeneous intrahepatic mass
Diagnosis: Hemangioma **(61)** with draining vein **(10)**
Differential diagnosis: Hyperechoic metastasis, hepatic tumors of other origin

Answer to Fig. 46.4 (Question 7):

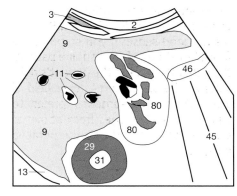

Imaging plane:
Right oblique subcostal plane
Organs:
Liver **(9)**, gallbladder **(80)**, kidney **(29)**
Significant finding: Inhomogeneous, poorly demarcated area along the caudal margin of the liver
Diagnosis: Cholecystitis with marked wall thickening **(80)**
Differential diagnosis: Parasitic involvement of liver or gallbladder, sludge, bowel content

Answer to Fig. 64.1 (Question 6):

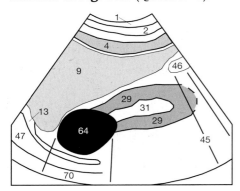

Imaging plane:
Intercostal plane of the right flank
Organs: Liver (9), kidney (29), lung
(47), bowel (46)
Structures:
Diaphragm (13), renal pelvis (31)
Significant finding:
Anechoic, spherical, sharply demarcated lesion (64) at the upper pole of
the right kidney, with distal acoustic
enhancement (70)
Diagnosis: Renal cyst (64)
Differential diagnosis:
Adrenal tumor with cystic components

Answer to Fig. 64.2 (Question 6):

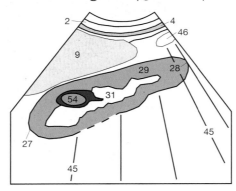

Imaging plane:
Intercostal plane of the right flank in
left lateral decubitus position
Organs: Liver (9), bowel (46) with
acoustic shadow (45), kidney (29)
Structures: External and internal
oblique muscles (4), upper and lower
poles of the kidney (27 and 28)
Significant finding: Ill-defined
hypoechoic lesion (54) in the renal
parenchyma (29) with mass effect
Diagnosis: Renal cell carcinoma
Differential diagnosis:
Renal lymphoma, metastasis,
hypertrophied column of Bertin,
hemorrhagic renal cyst

Answer to Fig. 64.3 (Question 7):

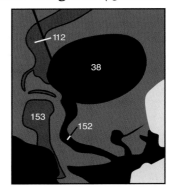

This voiding cystourethrogram was obtained during voiding (urethra = **152**)
with the patient in a slightly oblique
position to improve visualization of
both ureterovesical junctions to better
detect ureteral reflux.

The dark line extending cranially
from the bladder (**38**) is merely the
obliquely imaged cortex of the ilium
(**112**) projected on the femoral head
(**153**). Without the oblique positioning,
the normal ilium could be mistaken for
retrograde contrast filling of the ureter
in ureteral reflux.

Answer to Fig. 64.4 (Question 9):

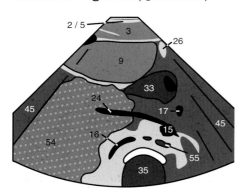

Imaging plane:
Transverse upper abdomen in an infant
Organs: Liver (9), pancreas (33)
Significant finding: Poorly demarcated
organs and large, inhomogeneous
tumor (54) in the right paravertebral
region. The tumor displaces the right
renal artery (24) anteriorly over a long
segment. Suspected lymph node
metastasis (55) between the aorta
(15) and lumbar vertebra (35)
Diagnosis:
Metastatic nephroblastoma (54)
Differential diagnosis:
Neuroblastoma of the right
sympathetic chain

Answer to Fig. 74.1 (Question 5):

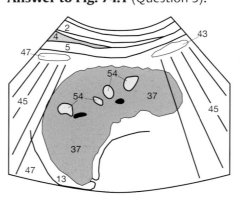

Imaging plane:
High plane of the left flank in the right
lateral decubitus position
Organs: Spleen (37), lung (47), colon
(43), diaphragm (13)
Significant finding:
Several sharply demarcated homogeneously hyperechoic lesions (54)
in the splenic parenchyma without a
hypoechoic rim
Diagnosis (rare finding):
Multiple splenic hemangiomas
Differential diagnosis:
Hyperechoic metastases, vasculitis
in systemic lupus erythematosus,
histiocytosis X

Answer to Fig. 92.1 (Question 7):

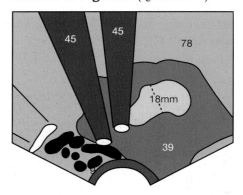

Imaging plane:
Endovaginal view of the uterus
Organs:
Uterus (39)
Significant finding:
Inhomogeneously hyperechoic
endometrium (78), widened to about
18 mm in a menopausal woman without hormonal therapy (see question).
Diagnosis:
Suspected endometrial carcinoma
Work-up: fractionated dilatation and
curettage for histologic evaluation

Answer to Question on page 42

The artifacts shown here are distal acoustic enhancement (70) and acoustic shadowing (45) behind the gallbladder (14). Fig. 39.3a shows two pathologic fluids:

68 = Ascites caudal to the diaphragm
69 = Pleural effusion cranial to the diaphragm
61 = Hemangioma with draining veins (10)

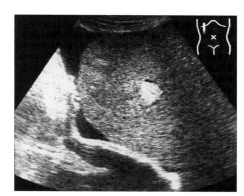

Fig. 125.1 a

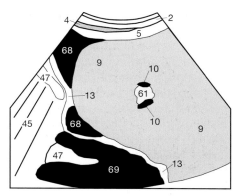

Fig. 125.1 b

Answer to Question on the Upper GI Series on page 66

Gravity causes the contrast medium (white) to collect in the more posterior fundus and in the pylorus and duodenum. The more anterior body of the stomach is easily evaluated on a double-contrast study. This distribution of contrast medium indicates that the patient is supine. If the examiner wants to evaluate the gastric fundus, the patient must be brought into the upright position or placed in an upright position to cause the contrast medium to flow out of the fundus.

To visualize the duodenal bulb on the right side, the patient must be placed in a left lateral position. Please remember that the upper GI series must be obtained in a fasting patient and that gastric peristalsis may need to be suppressed by medication (beware the side effects of intravenous scopolamine methylbromide!) to achieve a reliable result. It is advisable to tell patients beforehand to try not to burp and release the air produced by the effervescent powder. How else will they know?

Answer to Question on page 81

Fig. 77.2 illustrates the anatomic orientation on endovaginal images. The right edge of the image is posterior. The blood clot in the supine patient therefore appears on the right edge of the image in Fig. 81.3 as gravity brings it to rest in a posterior location.

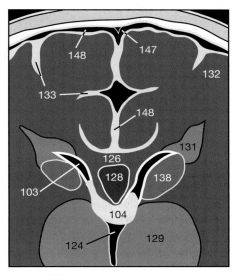

Fig. 125.2

Answer to Fig. 111.1 (Question 2):

Imaging plane:
Intracerebral coronal plane at the level of the foramina of Monro (144)
Structures:
Lateral ventricle (103), third ventricle (124), thalamus (129), cerebral sulci (133), choroid plexus (104), gray matter (132), periventricular white matter (131), corpus callosum (126), head of the caudate nucleus (138).
CSF spaces:

Interhemispheric fissure (146)	< 6 mm
Sinocortical width (147)	< 3 mm
Craniocortical width (148)	< 4 mm
Width of third ventricle (124)	< 10 mm
Width of lateral ventricle (anterior horn)	< 13 mm

Normal variant:
Cavum of the septum lucidum (128)

Acknowledgments

This revised and expanded edition could not have been realized without the support of numerous helpers. Since 1991, more than 11,000 course participants, scores of readers, and 150 course instructors have contributed to the continuing optimization of this workbook in systematic evaluations with feedback and constructive criticism. I wish to thank them all. I would like to express my particular gratitude to the following persons and institutions:

My special thanks go to Dipl. Designer Inger Wollziefer for the excellent graphical rendering of new sketches, the book's layout, and the supervision of production.

Ms. Wollziefer, Dr. Neuberger, and Ms. Tochtermann of Thieme Publishers and Druckerei Steinmeier have decisively contributed to ensuring that production went smoothly and efficiently. My heartfelt thanks to Aloka Deutschland GmbH, Siemens Health Care, Esaote Germany, and my colleagues C. F. Dietrich and C. Sproll, for providing images that demonstrate the importance of new techniques, and for their support in fundamental technical issues. Dr. Tatjana Reihs contributed most of the obstetric and gynecologic images, H.D. Matthiessen and J. Schaper valuable advice on hip screenings in newborn.

I cordially thank my wife Stefanie for her critical review and additional creative suggestions. I thank our two daughters Joana and Lea for the immense zest for living that they bring into our daily life, giving me the strength for book projects like this one. By way of thanks I have included images of both of them in this book (the question is where!).

Finally, I wish to pay tribute to all 32 present ultrasound instructors of our working group, their willingness to participate in intensive continuing education, and their indispensable contribution to the success of the entire project. Currently they include Dr. Nadine Abanador-Kamper, Jonathan Brück, Carina Büren, Kathrin Domagala, Anna Eisenhardt, Anna Falkowski, Dr. Arndt Giese, Ira Gabor, Lukas Goerdes, Katharina Groos-Sahr, Anna-Lena Hotze, Maike Huessmann, Anne Jaeckel, Dr. Lars Kamper, Sandra Malecha, David Mally, Golnessa Naeher, Kira Oesterwind, David Pullmann, Dr. Alexander Rosen, Dr. Ralf Rulands, Dr. Stefan Schmidt, Thomas Schmidt, Mirja Seisser, Gonxhe Shala, Katja Sievers, Benjamin Sigl, Richard Truse, and Kristina Wieferich.

Priv.-Doz. Matthias Hofer, M.D., MPH, MME
Diagnostic Radiologist
Director Medical Education Dept.
Heinrich Heine University Düsseldorf, Germany

More information on educational aspects concerning ultrasound courses

Ultrasound competencies play an important role in interdisciplinary all-day routine diagnostic algorithms. Therefore, in this field the quality management of educational activities has a significant impact on professional standards in medical school as well as in residency programs.

Colleagues who are interested to know more about our didactic approaches and training programs for ultrasound instructors, might want to have a look at several original articles:

Hofer M, Kamper L, Miese F, Kröpil P, Naujoks C, Heussen N.
Quality Indicators for the Conception and Didactics of Ultrasound Courses in Continuing Medical Education.
Ultraschall in Med. 2012; 33: 68–75

Hofer M, Kamper L, Sadlo M, Sievers K, Heussen N.
Evaluation of an OSCE-Assessment Tool for Abdominal Ultrasound Courses
Ultraschall in Med 2011; 32: 184–190
https://www.thieme-connect.de/DOI/DOI?10.1055/s-0029-1246049

Hofer M, Schiebel B, Hartwig HG, Mödder U.
Didactic skills trainings for ultrasound instructors.
Evaluation of the "Train-the-trainer" Program by the medical education pilot project.
Ultraschall in Med 2002; 23: 267–273

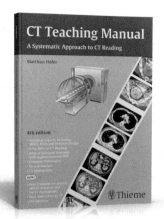
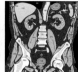
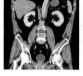
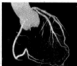

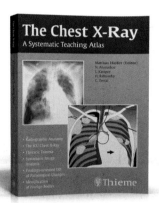
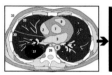
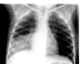
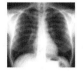
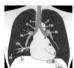
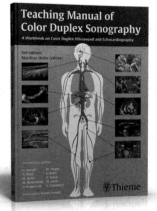
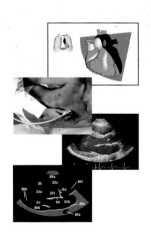
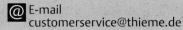
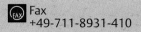
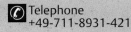
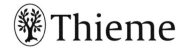
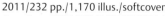